MAKING SENSE of
Lung Function Tests
Second edition

A hands-on guide

MAKING SENSE of
Lung Function Tests
Second edition

A hands-on guide

Jonathan Dakin, MD FRCP BSc Hons
Consultant Respiratory Physician
Royal Surrey County Hospital NHS Foundation Trust
Surrey, UK
Honorary Consultant Respiratory Physician
Portsmouth Hospitals NHS Trust
Hampshire, UK

Mark Mottershaw, BSc Hons MSc
Chief Respiratory Physiologist
Queen Alexandra Hospital
Portsmouth Hospitals NHS Trust
Hampshire, UK

Elena Kourteli, FRCA
Consultant Anaesthetist
St George's University Hospitals Foundation NHS Trust
London, UK

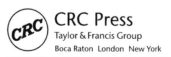

CRC Press
Taylor & Francis Group
Boca Raton London New York

CRC Press is an imprint of the
Taylor & Francis Group, an **informa** business

CRC Press
Taylor & Francis Group
6000 Broken Sound Parkway NW, Suite 300
Boca Raton, FL 33487-2742

© 2017 by Taylor & Francis Group, LLC
CRC Press is an imprint of Taylor & Francis Group, an Informa business

No claim to original U.S. Government works

Printed on acid-free paper

International Standard Book Number-13: 978-1-4822-4968-2 (Paperback)

Library of Congress Cataloging-in-Publication Data

A catalog record of this book is on file with the Library of Congress.

Visit the Taylor & Francis Web site at
http://www.taylorandfrancis.com

and the CRC Press Web site at
http://www.crcpress.com

Ὁ μεν βίος βραχὺς, ἡ δὲ τέχνη μακρὴ, ὁ δὲ καιρὸς ὀξὺς, ἡ δὲ πεῖρα σφαλερὴ, ἡ δὲ κρίσις χαλεπή.

Ἱπποκράτης

Life is short, science is long; opportunity is elusive, experiment is dangerous, judgement is difficult.

Hippocrates

Contents

Preface

Every doctor involved in acute medicine deals with blood gas or lung function data. Although a wealth of information lies therein, much of the content may be lost on the non-specialist. Frequently the information necessary for interpretation of basic data is buried deep in heavy specialist texts. This book sets out to unearth these gems and present them in a context and format useful to the frontline doctor. We accompany the clinical content with underlying physiology because we believe that for a little effort it offers worthwhile enlightenment. However, as life in clinical medicine is busy, we have placed the physiology in separate sections, so that those who want to get to the bottom line first can do so.

This book is not a technical manual, and details of performing laboratory test are kept to minimum to outline the physical requirements for successful compliance. Nor is it a reference manual for the specialist. The aim is to present information in an accessible way, suitable for those seeking a basic grounding in spirometry or blood gases, but also sufficiently comprehensive for readers completing specialist training in general or respiratory medicine.

ACKNOWLEDGEMENT

We wish to thank Warwick Hampden-Woodfall for essential IT backup.

Abbreviations

LUNG FUNCTION PARAMETERS

Ax	capacitance reactance area (Goldman triangle)
ERV	expiratory reserve volume
FEF	forced expiratory flow
FE_{NO}	fractional exhaled nitric oxide
FEV_1	forced expiratory volume within the first second
FRC	functional residual capacity
F_{res}	resonant frequency
FVC	forced vital capacity
G_{aw}	airway conductance
IC	inspiratory capacity
IRV	inspiratory reserve volume
IVC	inspiratory vital capacity
K_{CO}	transfer coefficient (measured using carbon monoxide)
MEP	maximal expiratory pressure
MIP	maximal inspiratory pressure
MVV	maximum voluntary ventilation
PEF	peak expiratory flow
PIF	peak inspiratory flow
R_5	total airway resistance
R_5–R_{20}	peripheral airway resistance
R_{20}	Central airway resistance
R_{aw}	airway resistance
RV	residual volume
sG_{aw}	specific airway conductance
Sniff P_{di}	sniff transdiaphragmatic pressure
SNIP	sniff inspiratory pressure
sR_{aw}	specific airway resistance
TLC	total lung capacity
TL_{CO}	transfer factor (measured using carbon monoxide)

V_A	alveolar volume
$\dot{V}_A$	minute volume of alveolar ventilation
VC	vital capacity
$\dot{V}_{CO_2}$	volume of CO_2 produced by the body per minute
V_D	dead space
$\dot{V}_E$	minute volume of ventilation
V_T	tidal volume
X_5	reactance

EXERCISE TESTING

6MWD	6 minute walk distance
6MWT	6 minute walk test
AT	anaerobic threshold
Borg	type of dyspnoea scale
BR	breathing reserve
$\dot{D}_{O_2}$	rate of oxygen delivery to the tissues
ESWT	endurance shuttle walk test
ISWT	incremental shuttle walk test
MVV	maximum voluntary ventilation per minute, usually extrapolated from a 15-second period of forced maximal breathing
RER	respiratory exchange ratio, given by $\dot{V}CO_2/\dot{V}O_2$
RPE	rating of perceived exertion
$\dot{V}_{CO_2}$	rate of oxygen carbon dioxide elimination by the lungs
$\dot{V}_E$	minute volume of ventilation
$\dot{V}_E/\dot{V}_{CO_2}$	ratio of minute ventilation to carbon dioxide elimination by the lungs (ventilatory equivalent for carbon dioxide)
$\dot{V}_E/\dot{V}_{O_2}$	ratio of minute ventilation to oxygen uptake by the lungs (ventilatory equivalent for oxygen)
$\dot{V}_{E_{cap}}$	maximum ventilatory capacity, usually derived from predictive equation using FEV_1
$\dot{V}_{O_2}$	rate of oxygen consumption
$\dot{V}_{O_{2MAX}}$	peak rate of oxygen consumption achieved during a maximal exercise test
$\dot{V}_{O_2}$ @ AT	oxygen consumption measured at the anaerobic threshold
$\dot{V}_{O_2}/HR$	oxygen consumption per heart beat (oxygen pulse)
WR	work rate (measured in watts, W)

Respiratory gas parameters

A–a	alveolar–arterial difference
ABG	arterial blood gas
$\dot{D}o_2$	rate of oxygen delivery to the tissues
HCO_3^-	bicarbonate
P_Aco_2	partial pressure of alveolar carbon dioxide
P_aco_2	partial pressure of arterial carbon dioxide
P_Ao_2	partial pressure of alveolar oxygen
P_ao_2	partial pressure of arterial oxygen
P_Io_2	partial pressure of inspired oxygen
P_vco_2	partial pressure of venous carbon dioxide
S_ao_2	oxyhaemoglobin saturation, measured directly by blood gas analysis
S_po_2	oxyhaemoglobin saturation, measured by peripheral pulse oximetry
$S_{\bar{v}}o_2$	mixed venous oxygen saturation, measured in blood from the pulmonary artery
$\dot{V}co_2$	rate of production of CO_2

Gases

CO	carbon monoxide
CO_2	carbon dioxide
He	helium
NO	nitric oxide
O_2	oxygen
ppb	parts per billion

Statistics

LLN	lower limit of normality
SD	standard deviation
SR	standard residual
ULN	upper limit of normality

Societies/Guidelines

ATS	American Thoracic Society
BTS	British Thoracic Society

ERS	European Respiratory Society
GINA	Global Initiative for Asthma
GOLD	Global Initiative for Chronic Obstructive Lung Disease
mMRC	Modified Medical Research Council (Dyspnoea Scale)
MRC	Medical Research Council (UK)
NICE	National Institute for Health and Care Excellence (UK)
SIGN	Scottish Intercollegiate Guidelines Network

DISEASES

ALS	amyotrophic lateral sclerosis
COPD	chronic obstructive pulmonary disease
ILD	interstitial lung disease
MND	motor neurone disease
OHS	obesity hypoventilation syndrome
OSA	obstructive sleep apnoea
RTA	renal tubular acidosis

UNITS

L	litre
min	minute
mmol	millimoles
mmol/L	millimoles per litre
s	second
SI	standard international (units)

MISCELLANEOUS

BODE	BMI, Obstruction, Dyspnoea and Exercise (index)
CK	creatinine kinase
CPAP	continuous positive airway pressure
CSF	cerebrospinal fluid
CT	computed tomography
ICS	inhaled corticosteroid
PEEP	positive end expiratory pressure
REM	rapid eye movement (sleep)

Expressions of normality

The percentage predicted has long been the favoured method of expressing lung function results amongst clinicians. It has the advantages of being easy to calculate and intuitive to understand. A test result which falls below 80% of the predicted value is often considered to be outside the range of natural variability and therefore abnormal, for a number of pulmonary function indices.

The percentage predicted is also used to grade severity of disease by comparing test results with a table of cut-off ranges. The number of categories and exact cut-offs are fairly arbitrary and vary between different respiratory societies. For example, one such table for identifying abnormal spirometry based on the FEV_1% predicted is shown in Table 1.1, modified from the American Thoracic Society (ATS)/European Respiratory Society (ERS) taskforce guidelines on interpretative strategies for lung function testing.[1] A similar classification is in common usage for peak flow readings in asthma (Table 2.1).

However, different lung function tests and indices have different degrees of natural variation within the population. For example, the transfer factor for carbon monoxide (TL_{CO}) has a wider inter-individual variability than many other lung function test values, and therefore a result which is 75% predicted may be well within the normal range. Moreover, this normal range may alter with age, so a value which is 75% of that predicted may be normal in the elderly, but warrant further investigation in the young.

This shortcoming has led clinical physiologists to favour the concept of the standard residual as a statistically more valid approach to identifying normal ranges. This method involves using standard deviations (SDs) to identify the upper and lower limits of normality (ULN and LLN respectively). Figure 1.1 shows a typical bell-shaped normal distribution curve and includes the percentage of values which lie within each SD (or Z score) and the mean. In a normal distribution, 95% of the population will record values within two SDs above or below the mean value.

The convention amongst physiologists is to use a value of 1.64 SDs to identify the ULN and LLN. This value is chosen because in a normal distribution

Table 1.1 Severity of airflow obstruction by FEV_1

Degree of severity	FEV_1% predicted
Normal	>80
Mild	70–79
Moderate	60–69
Moderately severe	50–59
Severe	35–49
Very severe	<35

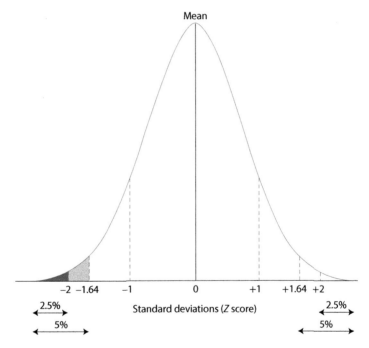

Figure 1.1 Normal distribution curve showing the percentage of a normal population who would fall 1.64 standard residuals beneath the mean. If the limit of normality is placed at 1.64 SDs below the mean, the healthy range encompasses 95% of the population.

90% of the population will fall within ±1.64 SDs of the mean, with 5% having 'supranormal' values above this range and 5% having 'abnormal' results below this range. However, there is no pathology associated with a supranormal value (with few exceptions such as measurements of airway resistances – see Chapter 8) and those fortunate individuals may be placed within the normal range, from a medical point of view. Therefore, the limit of –1.64 SDs below the mean identifies a 95% confidence limit, below which measurements are abnormal. The standard residual may be used to express the distance a result lies from the mean, and thereby grade the severity of abnormality, as shown in Table 1.2.

Table 1.2 Grade of severity by standard residual

Standard residual	Grade of severity
–1.64 or greater	Normal
–1.65 to –2.50	Mild
–2.50 to –3.50	Moderate
<–3.50	Severe

KEY POINTS

- The percentage of predicted is the most commonly used expression of normality, which is simple to calculate and intuitively understood. However, the cut-off for normality (e.g. <80%) is chosen arbitrarily and may result in under- or overdiagnosis of pathology.
- The use of standard residuals is more robust and provides a statistically valid method to identify values that fall below the limits of normal physiological variability. Usage of standard residuals is increasing and may ultimately replace the percentage predicted.

PART ①

TESTS OF AIRWAY FUNCTION AND MECHANICAL PROPERTIES

Peak expiratory flow

INTRODUCTION

Measurement of the peak expiratory flow (PEF) is one of the most convenient, economical, and commonly performed tests in the management of asthma. The test requires the simplest of measurement equipment and is straightforward to teach and perform.

TEST DESCRIPTION AND TECHNIQUE

The PEF is an easy test for most individuals to master but is dependent upon maximal effort, and so requires cooperation, coordination, and comprehension to produce repeatable and reliable results.

The test involves taking a forceful, full inspiration, immediately followed by short, maximal, explosive expiratory effort into the PEF meter. Expiration does not need to continue past the initial 'blast', as flow will quickly decline beyond this point.

The value recorded is usually the best of three efforts, each of which should be made with acceptable technique.

PITFALLS

- An isolated peak flow reading has limited value in diagnosing the cause of respiratory insufficiency, though it is helpful for monitoring known cases of asthma.
- The PEF can be 'cheated' by spitting into the meter like a blowpipe or pea-shooter. With practice, it is easy to blow the meter to the end of its scale with moderate effort using this technique.

PHYSIOLOGY OF TEST

PEF is the highest velocity of airflow that can be transiently achieved during a maximal expiration from total lung capacity. Because flow is a function of resistance, and the majority of resistance is encountered in the upper airways, the peak flow is an excellent indicator of large airway function.

In addition to airway resistance and effort, the PEF is also a function of lung volume and recoil, both of which increase as the lung is inflated. Therefore, measurements should be made after a full inspiration.

NORMAL VALUES

Normal values for PEF are commonly read from a nomogram, similar to that shown in Figure 2.1.[2] Note that values at all ages are directly related to height, but that males have higher values than females of the same height and age.

These nomograms are constructed from regression equations derived from large population studies. The most commonly used regression equations in Europe are those calculated from the European Community of Coal and Steelworkers (ECCS) study.[3] The equations for calculation of predicted normal values for PEF for males and females are as follows:

Males: PEF $(L \cdot s^{-1})$ = (6.14 × height) − (0.043 × age) + 0.15

Females: PEF $(L \cdot s^{-1})$ = (5.50 × height) − (0.030 × age) − 1.11

PEAK FLOW VARIABILITY IN THE DIAGNOSIS OF ASTHMA

The key to assessment of asthma is a careful history, which in many cases will allow a reasonably certain clinical diagnosis. Nonetheless, as treatment may be required over many years, it is important even in relatively clear cases to try to obtain objective support for the diagnosis where possible.[4]

Confirmation of a diagnosis of asthma hinges upon demonstration of airflow obstruction, varying over short periods of time.

A period of monitoring may be helpful by identifying diurnal variation, which is a hallmark of asthma, to add weight to a diagnosis in uncertain cases. During a period of monitoring, peak flow should be measured at least twice per day, morning and night, and recorded on a peak flow chart similar to that shown in Figure 2.2.

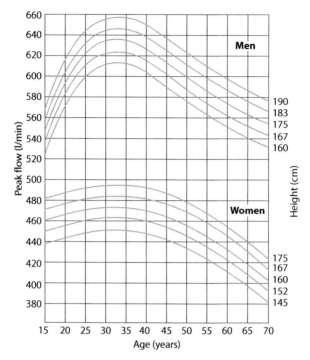

Figure 2.1 Peak flow nomogram showing normal peak flow values for males and females by age and height. During childhood, peak flows are similar for boys and girls of the same height. During adolescence, the two curves diverge, so that the predicted peak flow is greater for a short man than for a tall woman. Hence, the two sets of curves have no overlap. (Reproduced from Gregg I and Nunn AJ, *Br Med J*, 3, 282–284, 1973. With permission from the BMJ Publishing Group.)

Daily diurnal PEF variability is calculated from twice daily PEF as

$$\frac{\text{Each day's highest } - \text{ Same day's lowest}}{\text{Mean of that day's highest and lowest}}$$

The above equation should be applied to the highest and lowest results for each day, to produce a daily percentage variability over the period of monitoring. All of the percentages should then be averaged, over at least 1 week.[4]

The threshold of significance of diurnal PEF variability depends upon how many readings are taken per day, as the more readings are taken, the

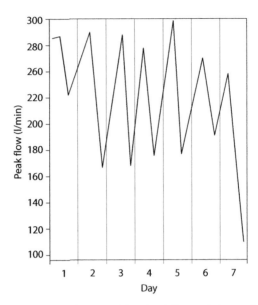

Figure 2.2 Diurnal peak flow variability. Peak flow only has a slight diurnal variability in normal subjects, with the lowest values usually seen in the early hours of the morning. The wide variation in this asthmatic is seen during very poor control, with a final dangerous deterioration.

greater the likelihood that the true daily maximum and minimum PEF will be identified. Thus, if two daily readings are taken (morning and night) then a variability of 10% is significant, whereas a variability of 20% is required where four or more readings are recorded. A four-time daily monitoring schedule would be difficult for most patients to maintain.

Notwithstanding the above, the sensitivity of peak flow variability monitoring for diagnosing asthma is not high, at around 25%.[4] Moreover, patients with other causes of obstructive lung disease may also show some degree of peak flow variability, reducing the specificity of variability monitoring as a diagnostic test. Greater sensitivity may be gained by monitoring peak flow for a 2-week period prior to treatment, followed by 2 weeks after commencement. However, the time required to calculate this is not insignificant.

Electronic peak flow devices are available which record the time at which readings are made and automatically calculate the variability. Use of such devices ensures that readings are made at appropriate times.

Very wide variability in daily PEF readings is a feature of poorly controlled or brittle asthma. Brittle asthmatics may exhibit PEF variability of 40% or more. Large variability in PEF is also observed in the recovery phase of acute severe asthma and indicates ongoing lability. A patient who has been admitted to hospital with acute asthma should not be discharged until the diurnal variability in PEF is less than 25%.

Peak flow monitoring is an essential tool in the diagnosis of occupational asthma. The portability of the peak flow metre enables convenient serial readings to be made during the working day, so that the effects of occupational exposure may be measured at the time of contact with the suspected sensitising agent.

ASSESSMENT AND MANAGEMENT OF ASTHMA

Asthmatics should have their own self-management plan to guide escalation of treatment, based on any deterioration of peak flow and clinical symptoms. All patients with severe asthma should have their own peak flow metre and a familiarity of their own range of values.[4]

The PEF reading gives an objective and early warning signal of the need to increase therapy or seek medical intervention.

A sudden deterioration in the peak flow of an asthmatic may occur during exacerbations and be a premonitory warning of such. In a patient suffering an acute exacerbation of asthma, a PEF of less than 75% of their normal best value (or the patient's predicted, whichever is less) suggests a moderate exacerbation. A PEF of less than 50% of best or predicted is a feature of acute severe asthma. A patient with a PEF of this order, particularly when it persists after bronchodilator therapy, should be admitted to hospital. A PEF of less than 33% of a patient's normal best or predicted value indicates life-threatening asthma.

Severity of acute asthma, as gauged by PEF, is summarised in Table 2.1.

Table 2.1 Severity of acute asthma by peak expiratory flow

Severity of acute asthma exacerbation	% of normal best or predicted
Moderate exacerbation	50%–75%
Acute severe exacerbation	33%–50%
Life-threatening exacerbation	<33%

PITFALL

Diurnal variation may be missed if PEF is not measured first thing in the morning, prior to bronchodilator therapy.

KEY POINTS

- Diurnal variability in PEF is a hallmark of asthma.
- Peak flow measurements are essential for assessing the severity of acute asthma.
- Peak flow variability monitoring may be useful in the management of some asthmatics.
- Peak flow variability monitoring may be useful in the diagnosis of asthma.
- There are many causes of a low PEF other than asthma.
- Peak flow monitoring is requisite for assessment of suspected occupational asthma.

3

Spirometry and the flow–volume loop

INTRODUCTION

Spirometry is one of the most fundamental tests of pulmonary function. On the basis of this measurement, obstructive pulmonary pathology may be diagnosed and restrictive disease suspected. The pivotal role of spirometry makes this the most important chapter of this book.

The spirogram is a plot of volume against time, taken as a subject breathes out after a full inspiration.

The flow–volume loop is an alternative way of looking at the same data. On the flow–volume loop, flow is plotted against volume, without reference to time. This is a less intuitive representation, but once familiar lends itself to pattern recognition of a number of abnormalities which are less apparent on the spirogram. Figure 3.1 shows the appearance of normal spirometry, represented on both volume–time and flow–volume axes.

MEASURED INDICES AND KEY DEFINITIONS

Table 3.1 shows the commonly used parameters which are measured during spirometry.

TEST DESCRIPTION AND TECHNIQUE

Spirometry has historically been measured using a mechanical wedge-bellows spirometer, with the analogue trace depicted on a volume–time graph. Flow–volume loops require electronic processing, so that most devices in current usage are digital and capable of displaying results as either a spirogram or a flow–volume loop.

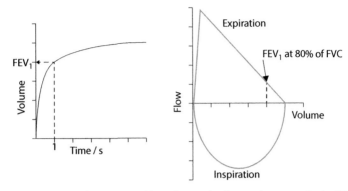

Figure 3.1 Normal spirometry. Note that on the flow–volume graph, the FEV_1 cannot actually be read from the graph (as there is no time axis), but is shown for illustration purposes. Similarly, there is no way to assess expiratory time on the flow–volume trace.

Table 3.1 Parameters measured at spirometry

Abbrev.	Index	Unit	Definition/comment
FVC	Forced vital capacity	L	The volume of the lungs that can be expired with *maximal force* following a full inspiration from total lung capacity.
VC	Vital capacity	L	The maximum volume that can be expired during a *comfortably paced expiration* to residual volume. (May also be described as a relaxed or slow VC to distinguish from the FVC.)
FEV_1	Forced expiratory volume in 1 second	L	The volume that can be expired in the first second of a maximal FVC.
FEV_1/FVC or FEV_1/VC	FEV_1 ratio	%	The FEV_1 divided by whichever is the larger of the VC or FVC.

(Continued)

Table 3.1 (*Continued*) Parameters measured at spirometry

Abbrev.	Index	Unit	Definition/comment
PEF	Peak expiratory flow	L/min	Maximum expiratory flow, see Chapter 2.
PIF	Peak inspiratory flow	L/min	Maximum inspiratory flow measured whilst recording a flow–volume loop.

The archetypal volume–time graph (spirogram) still adds value, as the output from a wedge-bellows spirometer is a direct analogue transmission of patient effort, without intervening electronic signal processing. Therefore, this provides the gold standard in terms of data resolution.

However, the flow–volume loop lends itself to pattern recognition of a wider variety of ventilatory defects, with deficiencies in test performance easier to identify. Therefore, the flow–volume loop is considered a more informative graphical representation of airflow data by most clinicians and physiologists.

Pre-test instructions should be observed to standardise spirometry results. These include abstaining from smoking, drinking alcohol, large meals, and strenuous exercise for a suitable period before measurement, as well as usually the use of any prescribed bronchodilator medication.

The relaxed vital capacity (VC) is performed by taking a maximal inspiration, followed by a complete expiration at a comfortable pace into the measuring equipment. This test is repeated by a more forceful maximal inspiration, then a maximal, explosive, and complete exhalation to record FEV_1 and forced vital capacity (FVC). If the equipment is capable of producing a flow–volume loop, the manoeuvre ends with a subsequent forced inspiration back to total lung capacity (TLC).

There are contraindications to spirometry, due to the changes in intrathoracic pressure and haemodynamics which occur during what is effectively a Valsalva manoeuvre.[5,6] In the main, these are common sense and usually relative contraindications, the decision regarding suitability often depending on an analysis of risk versus benefit. A recent myocardial infarction or pneumothorax would predictably usually constitute an absolute contraindication, as would a cerebral aneurysm, due to the unopposed increase in cerebral vascular pressure associated with Valsalva-type manoeuvres. The main contraindications are shown in Table 3.2.

Table 3.2 Contraindications to performing spirometry

Contraindication	Comment/example
Haemoptysis of unknown origin	Forced manoeuvre may exacerbate. The possibility of tuberculosis (TB) may be concerning for infection risk.
Pneumothorax	
Recent myocardial infarction	
Suspected untreated pulmonary embolism	
Aortic or cerebral aneurysms	Danger of rupture due to increased thoracic pressure.
Recent eye surgery	Cataract.
Acute disease which interferes with test	Vomiting, acute dyspnoea.
Recent surgery of thorax or abdomen	

Spirometry can be performed by most individuals, but like measurements of peak flow is dependent on comprehension, coordination, and cooperation for reliable results to be obtained. Referrals for spirometry should take this into account.

PHYSIOLOGY OF TESTS

RESTRICTIVE AND OBSTRUCTIVE DEFECTS

The FEV_1 and FVC are both volumetric measurements. However, as a volume expired *within a set time*, FEV_1 is also a reflection of average *airflow* over the first 1 second. Therefore, FEV_1 reflects the *speed of emptying of the lungs*. The FEV_1/FVC expression may be considered as a ratio of airflow/lung volume.

RESTRICTIVE DEFECTS

The maximal FVC that an individual can achieve is first dependent upon the ability of the respiratory musculature to fully inflate the lungs, against the combined elastance of the lungs and chest wall. This elastance is the reciprocal of compliance and is the 'springiness', which tends to return the lung volume to functional residual capacity (FRC), the natural resting point of the combined mechanical system (see 'Functional residual capacity' in Chapter 7).

Second, the FVC is dependent upon the ability of the lungs to empty during expiration to their residual volume (RV) (see 'Residual volume' in Chapter 7).

Restrictive processes are those which limit lung expansion, so reducing the TLC. Broadly, a restrictive process may be caused by disease of the chest wall, respiratory musculature, pleura, or the lung parenchyma, any of which may limit pulmonary expansion. Table 3.3 lists a variety of examples.

Reduction of FVC or VC suggests the presence of a restrictive defect. However, reduction of FVC may alternatively be caused by gas trapping in small airways during expiration. Under these circumstances, the RV may expand at the expense of FVC, but within the same TLC (Figure 7.5). Reduced VC in this scenario reflects small airways disease rather than failure of expansion *and is not a true restrictive defect.*

Therefore, measurement of static lung volumes (FRC, TLC, and RV) is required to make the distinction between a true restrictive defect

Table 3.3 Causes of a restrictive defect

Category	Examples
Interstitial lung disease	Idiopathic pulmonary fibrosis
	Sarcoidosis
	Hypersensitivity pneumonitis (extrinsic allergic alveolitis)
	Asbestosis
Loss of pulmonary volume	Post-lobectomy/pneumonectomy
	Atelectasis
Intrathoracic space occupying lesion	Large hiatus hernia
	Gross cardiomegaly
Pleural disease	Diffuse asbestos-related pleural thickening
	Pleural thickening post-empyema
	Pleural effusion
Chest wall disorder	Kyphoscoliosis
	Ankylosing spondylitis
	Severe obesity
	Scleroderma 'hide bound chest'
Neuromuscular disorder	Motor neurone disease
	Guillain–Barré
	Diaphragmatic palsy
	Muscular dystrophy
	Polymyositis

and reduction of FVC due to gas trapping. Only a reduction of TLC is specific for the diagnosis of a restrictive condition. Only in one half of cases is a reduction of FVC due to reduction of TLC. Moreover, a reduction of FVC which occurs in the context of an obstructive defect is rarely due to a restrictive process.

OBSTRUCTIVE DEFECTS

As a reflection of *airflow*, the FEV_1 is determined by airway function and is susceptible to the effects of airways disease, such as asthma and chronic obstructive pulmonary disease (COPD). These processes are described as obstructive.

However, the airflow generated in expiration is also a reflection of the volume of the lung which is driving that expiration. Therefore, any condition causing a loss of FVC also causes a proportionate reduction of airflow. Under these circumstances, a normal FEV_1/FVC ratio is preserved. By contrast, an obstructive disease reduces FEV_1 disproportionately, so that the FEV_1/FVC ratio is also reduced.

KEY POINTS

- Reduction of the FEV_1 ratio defines the obstructive state.
- Reduction of FVC may raise a suspicion of a restrictive disorder, but definition of restriction hinges upon reduction of TLC.

MAXIMUM EXPIRATORY FLOWS

A key characteristic of spirometry is reproducibility. This reproducibility is due to limitation of the maximum value of FEV_1 by the mechanical properties of the airways, rather than effort. Beyond a certain threshold of adequate effort, any further increase in the value of FEV_1 is dependent upon the characteristics of the lungs and airways, rather than force applied.

At the beginning of a forced expiration, air leaving the lungs originates from the large airways, in which cartilaginous rings support the airway and resist compression. However, air which subsequently leaves the lungs originates from smaller airways, which lack this cartilaginous support. Therefore, these airways themselves are narrowed by the compressive force of the chest wall upon the lungs during a forced expiration (Figure 3.2). This 'dynamic

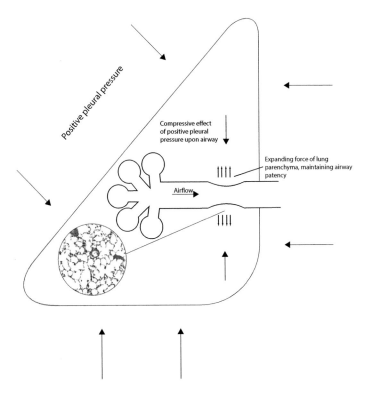

Figure 3.2 Dynamic airway collapse. Changes in airway pressure during respiratory manoeuvres, showing dynamic airway compression on forced expiration. Positive pleural pressure creates positive alveolar pressure to drive expiration. Air is expelled down the pressure gradient to the airway opening. However, at the same time, positive pleural pressure is applied to the airway, which limits flow downstream of the alveoli. Patency of airways then depends upon the elastic recoil of the tissues in which they are embedded.

airway compression' is the principle rate limiter of airflow during the latter period of expiration, rather than effort.

In normal lungs, it is the elasticity or recoil of the healthy lung parenchyma which holds open the small airways during expiration, by tethering them in an open position. By contrast, emphysematous lungs lack this support, so that small airways collapse early in expiration due to the application of positive pleural pressure (see Figures 3.3 and 3.4).[7] (See also Chapter 8 for more detailed discussion.)

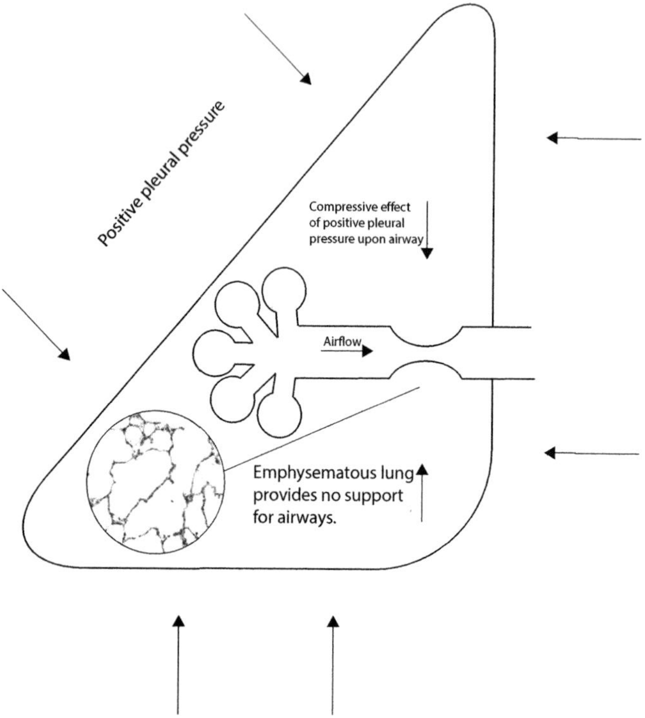

Figure 3.3 Dynamic airway collapse in emphysema. The emphysematous lung provides neither tethering nor expansive force to the airway during expiration. Therefore, the positive pleural pressure acts to close the airways during a forced expiration, reducing FEV_1.

NORMAL VALUES

Results of spirometry are compared with regression equations derived from population studies. Historically, the lower limit of normality of an FVC (or VC) has been defined as 80% of the predicted mean value. A more robust approach is to express these values in terms of the standard residual, with a lower limit of normality at 1.64 residuals below the mean (see discussion in Chapter 1).

The lower limit of normality of the FEV_1 ratio has been fixed at 0.7, by a number of airways disease guidelines.[8,9] This definition is the subject of some controversy, as the FEV_1/FVC ratio naturally declines with age, so that the

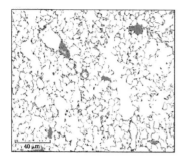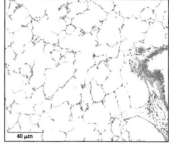

Figure 3.4 Pathology of emphysema. Normal histological appearance of lung parenchyma on the left, showing alveoli. The micrograph on the right shows emphysema, with widespread loss of alveoli. The destruction of alveolar units reduces lung elasticity as well as gas-exchanging surface area. (From Morris DG and Sheppard D, *Physiology*, 21, 396–403, 2006. With permission.)

lower limit of normality falls through 0.7 by the age of 47. Therefore, a fixed threshold of 0.7 for the diagnosis of airway obstruction is overinclusive for the healthy elderly population, and insensitive for the young.[10] The authors would strongly encourage use of the lower limit of normality of the FEV_1 ratio based upon standard residuals for the age of the patient, rather than 0.7.

The predicted value of FEV_1/FVC for a male of 40 years and average height (175 cm) is 4.1/5 L. For a female aged 40 and of average height (161 cm), the predicted values of FEV_1/FVC are 2.8/3.2. The lower limit of normality of the FEV_1 ratio for males at the age of 20 is 0.83, falling to 0.63 by the age of 70. The FEV_1 ratio is not affected greatly by height.

ASSESSMENT OF SEVERITY OF OBSTRUCTION

Importantly, the value of the FEV_1 (percent predicted) is used to assess severity of an obstructive defect, rather than the FEV_1 ratio. The FEV_1 ratio is not used for severity assessment, because it may be relatively preserved in patients whose FVC is also reduced, as frequently occurs in the presence of obstruction, due to gas trapping (see 'Reduction of FEV_1 and FVC').

The GOLD guideline for management of patients with COPD[8] provides a scheme for identifying the severity of airflow limitation, defined according to the FEV_1 ratio and the FEV_1 % predicted (Table 3.4).

The guidelines recommend that those subjects whose FEV_1 ratio is <0.7 despite an FEV_1 >80% should only be diagnosed with COPD if

Table 3.4 GOLD classification of airflow limitation in COPD

FEV$_1$ ratio	FEV$_1$% predicted	Severity
>0.7	>80%	Normal
<0.7	≥80%	Stage 1 – Mild
<0.7	50%–79%	Stage 2 – Moderate
<0.7	30%–49%	Stage 3 – Severe
<0.7	<30%	Stage 4 – Very severe

symptomatic. Importantly, there is no one lung function test which defines COPD, diagnosis of which is made on the basis of a number of clinical and physiological features. The values of FEV$_1$ used in the definitions are those measured after administration of bronchodilator, though formal reversibility testing is not required to make the diagnosis.

KEY POINT

Whereas the FEV$_1$ ratio is used to define the presence of an obstructive defect, the FEV$_1$ (percent predicted) is used to describe the severity.

MID-EXPIRATORY FLOWS

Mid-expiratory flow values are additional parameters which may be generated on the report of a spirogram or flow–volume loop. These are defined as the forced expiratory flow (FEF) generated after a specified percentage of a patient's VC has been expired:

- FEF$_{25}$ – maximum achievable flow after 25% of VC has been expired.
- FEF$_{25-75}$ – mean flow between 25% and 75% of VC.

Likewise, the FEF$_{50}$ and the FEF$_{75}$ are the FEF at the points when 50% and 75% of the VC have been expired. The FEF$_{25-75}$ was formerly known as the maximal mid-expiratory flow.

These indices have been credited with providing a better insight into small airway disease than the traditional indices of FEV$_1$ or peak flow. Although FEFs are very sensitive to disease, they are not specific and may be 'abnormal' in many asymptomatic and healthy individuals. Therefore, they are not widely quoted nor utilised in clinical practice.

FVC VERSUS VC

In health or disease, the VC is generally somewhat greater than the FVC, for reasons which are poorly understood. The disparity between the two measurements tends to be greater in patients with airflow obstruction. Thus, the difference between the FVC and VC provides an additional index of gas trapping.

Therefore, use of the VC rather than the FVC as the denominator of the FEV_1 ratio may result in a lower FEV_1 ratio, and so is more sensitive in the detection of an obstructive defect (e.g. in the diagnosis of COPD or asthma). Most of the airways disease guidelines specify the use of FVC,[4,9,11] or where use of either FVC or VC is suggested,[8] no preference is stated. Regardless of which denominator is chosen, the lower limit of normality of the FEV_1 ratio is set at 0.7.

By contrast, the American Thoracic Society (ATS)/European Respiratory Society (ERS) guidelines for interpretation of lung function[1] stand alone in suggesting that the greater of FVC or VC should be used as the denominator of the FEV_1 ratio, and therefore in defining an obstructive disorder. The authors prefer this definition, which seems more rational. Moreover, these guidelines also recommend an age-specific lower limit for the FEV_1 ratio, reflecting the natural decline of this value in the healthy elderly population.

PATTERNS OF ABNORMALITY

The two major patterns of intrathoracic abnormality which may be suggested by spirometry are obstructive and restrictive, although both may coexist. Extrathoracic abnormalities may also be identified, particularly by reference to the shape of the flow–volume loop.

OBSTRUCTIVE SPIROMETRY

The more commonly encountered spirometric defect is the obstructive pattern, signifying airflow limitation, and increased airway resistance. The primary abnormality in obstructive spirometry is a reduction in the FEV_1 ratio. The FEV_1 ratio is the most sensitive marker of obstruction, as the FEV_1 may be reduced, but still lie within normal limits in a subject whose FVC lies above average.

Figure 3.5 shows typical changes to the spirogram and flow–volume loop of a patient with mild obstructive airways disease. Note the characteristic 'scalloping' of the expiratory curve of the flow–volume loop, indicating that some lung units have increased airway resistance and empty at a different,

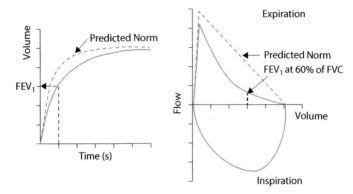

Figure 3.5 Spirometry showing mild airflow limitation. Spirometric traces showing mild airflow limitation, with a lower FEV$_1$ on the volume–time graph and scalloping of the expiratory flow–volume trace. Note that the position of the FEV$_1$ (again shown only for illustration) moves to the left on the volume axis of the flow–volume graph.

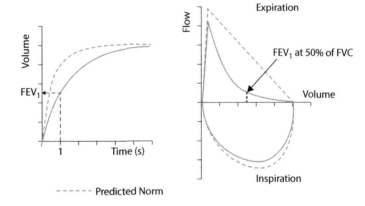

Figure 3.6 Spirometry showing moderate airflow limitation. Spirometric traces showing moderate airflow limitation. Note the increased scalloping and further leftward move of the FEV$_1$ position on the flow–volume x-axis.

slower rate to normal airways. Figures 3.6 and 3.7 show typical changes for obstructive spirometry classified as moderate and severe, respectively. The spirometry trace shown in Figure 3.7 is so distinctive of emphysema that it is virtually diagnostic.

This pattern arises from the reduction of recoil, secondary to the loss of distal lung parenchyma which characterises emphysema, so that airways

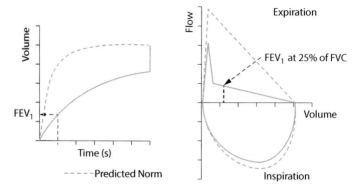

Figure 3.7 'Church spire' flow–volume loop showing severe airflow limitation. Severe airflow limitation with a 'church spire' flow–volume trace characteristic of emphysema. Note also that expiratory time exceeds the maximal time of the x-axis of the volume–time trace.

collapse as soon as intrathoracic pressure is increased by a forced expiratory effort (see 'Maximum expiratory flows').

RESTRICTIVE SPIROMETRY

The restrictive defect is defined by a reduction of TLC. Although TLC cannot be measured using spirometry, the FVC parallels TLC throughout many disease processes, making it a useful surrogate.

KEY POINT

An obstructive defect is defined spirometrically by an FEV_1 ratio below the lower limit of normality, sometimes taken as 0.7. Although a restrictive defect may be *suspected* by reduction of FVC (or VC), it is defined by reduction of TLC to below the lower limit of normality (see 'Restrictive defects' in 'Physiology of tests').

By contrast to the obstructive pattern, the FEV_1 ratio is preserved (or may be increased) in restrictive disorders. However, the absolute values of the FEV_1 are reduced along with the VC.

Three different restrictive patterns may be seen on flow–volume loops. In the first, the expiratory portion of the flow–volume loop looks like a pointy 'wizard's hat' (see Figure 3.8). This is typical of interstitial lung diseases where fibrotic changes to the lung parenchyma traction open the airways,

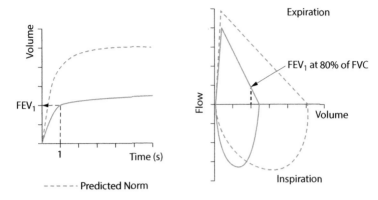

Figure 3.8 'Wizard hat' flow–volume loop showing ventilatory restriction. 'Wizard hat' restrictive spirometry with reduced VC, reduced FEV$_1$ and elevated FEV$_1$ ratio due to reduced compliance.

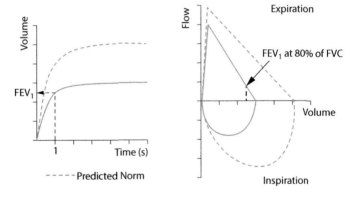

Figure 3.9 Restrictive spirometry with normal flow–volume loop morphology. Restrictive spirometry with a normal looking spirometry trace which is reduced in magnitude.

increasing the speed of lung emptying, as well as reducing compliance and preventing appropriate inflation.

The second pattern is a normal-shaped trace, which is simply reduced in magnitude (see Figure 3.9). This may be seen when TLC is reduced in the absence of pulmonary disease, for example in the presence of a pleural effusion or post-pulmonary resection.

A third pattern may be seen in subjects with respiratory muscle weakness (Figure 3.10). A rather rounded expiratory flow–volume trace may be seen,

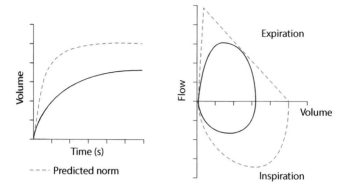

Figure 3.10 Restrictive spirometry seen in respiratory muscle weakness. The maximum flow appears rather later on the flow–volume loop. The flow falls off rather abruptly thereafter, with a convex shape, by contrast to the concavity seen in an obstructed trace.

with a maximum flow which occurs rather later, due to the subject's inability to create an explosive muscular effort on expiration.

REDUCTION OF FEV_1 AND FVC

Confusingly, obstructive airways disease may also be associated with a reduction in VC. This is caused by gas trapping within the RV, so that RV increases at the expense of VC, whilst the overall TLC (RV + VC) remains unchanged (see explanation in the section 'Restrictive defects' in 'Physiology of tests' and Figure 7.5).

Therefore, this is not a true restrictive defect, as it is caused by airways disease rather than impairment of expansion. Access to more detailed lung function measurement would be required to elucidate the true nature of this combination. This scenario is seen commonly in both asthma and COPD, occurring in up to 40% of cases of obstruction.[12]

MIXED OBSTRUCTIVE/RESTRICTIVE DEFECT

A genuine combined defect may occur when obstructive and restrictive pulmonary pathologies coexist. For example, many patients with idiopathic pulmonary fibrosis have also smoked in the past and have coexisting emphysema. Nonetheless, a genuine combined defect is uncommon. This is in part due to the abnormally stiff lung parenchyma that characterises interstitial lung disease, which tends to hold open the airways in expiration, so that expiratory flow remains normal, even in those with radiological evidence of advanced emphysema, when it coexists with pulmonary fibrosis. Occasionally, pulmonary sarcoidosis may cause both airways disease and interstitial fibrosis, giving a combined defect.

NON-SPECIFIC VENTILATORY DEFECT

A further scenario may arise in which the FVC is reduced in isolation, with preservation of both the FEV_1 ratio and TLC, i.e. in the absence of both obstruction and true restriction. This has been termed a non-specific ventilatory defect.[13] As above, the RV has increased at the expense of the FVC, within the same TLC envelope. This may be due to airways disease in asthma or bronchiolitis, but centred upon small airways and causing no demonstrable obstructive defect.

Table 3.5 summarises the changes in the major indices of spirometry for obstructive, restrictive, and combined pulmonary disorders.

Table 3.5 Changes in common indices with different spirometric defects

Defect	FEV_1	FVC or VC	FEV_1 ratio	Examples
Normal	>80% predicted >LLN SR ≥ −1.64	>80% predicted >LLN	>70% >LLN SR ≥ −1.64	Asthma when asymptomatic
		SR ≥ −1.64		
Obstructive	Usually ↓	↔ or ↓	↓	COPD Asthma Bronchiolitis
Restrictive	↓	↓	↔ or ↑	Pulmonary fibrosis Sarcoidosis Scoliosis Motor neurone disease
Combined	↓	↓	↓	Sarcoidosis Combined pulmonary fibrosis and emphysema

Abbreviation: LLN, Lower Limit of Normality

This schema may be further simplified by focusing upon the FEV_1 ratio and FVC, as shown in Table 3.6. Note the simplicity of this approach and unique pattern of change in each distinct type of abnormal spirometry.

Table 3.6 Simplified interpretation of spirometry

Spirometry	FVC_1% predicted	FEV_1 ratio
Normal	>80 (↔)	>70 (↔)
Obstructive	>80 (↔)	<70 (↓)
Restrictive	<80 (↓)	>70 (↔)
Combined	<80 (↓)	<70 (↓)

LARGE AIRWAYS OBSTRUCTION

The flow–volume loop is extremely sensitive in detecting the presence of upper airway lesions, which may not be obvious from the simple spirogram. Anatomically this includes all airways from the carina to the oropharynx. Three patterns of major airway obstruction can be observed on the flow–volume loop. These are fixed, variable intrathoracic and variable extrathoracic. The shape of the flow–volume loop can therefore not only indicate the presence of upper airway flow limitation, but also the likely anatomical location of the lesion.

Examples of conditions producing major airway obstruction include retrosternal goitre, vocal cord paralysis, and laryngeal and tracheal tumours.

FIXED UPPER AIRWAY OBSTRUCTION

This defect indicates a lesion anywhere in the upper airway, which limits flow equally on inspiration and expiration. The typical pattern of this defect is shown in Figure 3.11 and displays a 'decapitation' or flattening of the normal shape of the flow–volume loop on both the inspiratory and expiratory phases.

VARIABLE EXTRATHORACIC OBSTRUCTION

The extrathoracic upper airways include all airways superior to the thoracic inlet, the superior border of the thoracic cavity.

Variable upper airway obstruction occurs when one of the phases of the breathing cycle (either inspiratory or expiratory) is compromised to a greater extent than the other. An extrathoracic obstruction compromises inspiration to a greater extent than expiration, as negative pressure within the extrathoracic airway tends to collapse the lumen.

The characteristic pattern seen on a flow–volume trace in this situation is a flattening or 'squaring' of the *inspiratory* loop, with the expiratory phase largely unaffected (see Figure 3.12). Numerical reference to the peak *inspiratory* flow will quantify the defect, although the pattern of the inspiratory loop is instantly recognisable. Results such as those shown in Figure 3.12 suggest a significant upper airway obstruction such as that caused by the tracheal tumour shown in Figure 3.13.

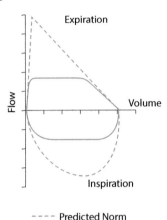

Figure 3.11 Flow–volume loop showing fixed upper airway obstruction. There is marked reduction of both the peak inspiratory and peak expiratory flow (PEF).

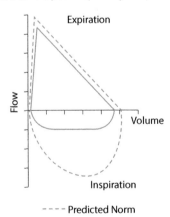

Figure 3.12 Variable extrathoracic obstruction. Reduction of the peak inspiratory flow causes flattening of the inspiratory portion of the flow–volume loop.

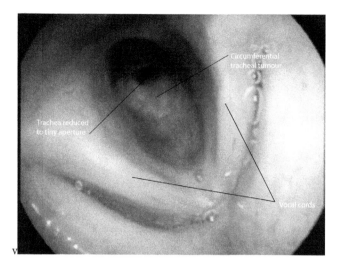

Figure 3.13 Bronchoscopic view of tracheal stenosis. Tumour occluding a substantial proportion of the upper airway, causing variable extrathoracic obstruction.

VARIABLE INTRATHORACIC OBSTRUCTION

The intrathoracic portion of the upper airway extends from the carina superiorly to the thoracic inlet. These airways are subject to the compressive effect of positive intrathoracic pressure during *expiration*, further compromising any stenosis caused by luminal obstruction. Thus, variable obstruction in these airways is revealed on the expiratory phase of the flow–volume loop. The pattern produced is different to that caused by airflow limitation in the smaller airways. The usual expiratory curve is somewhat decapitated, with the inspiratory phase relatively unaffected (see Figures 3.14 and 3.15).

CLINICAL PEARLS

- In those with an obstructive defect, the reduction in the value of peak expiratory flow (PEF) is relatively less than that of FEV_1, making FEV_1 a better index, particularly in COPD. This is seen on the flow–volume loop in emphysema, where the peak flow remains high (the tip of the 'church spire'), despite collapse of expiratory flow thereafter (Figure 3.7).

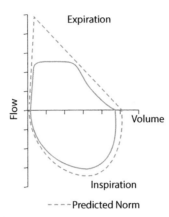

Expiration

Flow

Volume

Inspiration

- - - - Predicted Norm

Figure 3.14 Variable intrathoracic obstruction. There is marked reduction of the PEF, causing flattening or 'decapitation' of the flow–volume loop. Major airway obstruction can also be identified on a volume–time graph and produces a pattern known as a straight line spirogram shown in Figure 3.15. However, this may be mistaken for an incomplete expiration or a leak, and these defects are much easier to identify on a flow–volume graph.

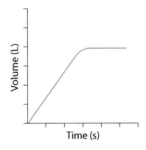

Volume (L)

Time (s)

Figure 3.15 Straight line spirogram. This pattern of abnormality is another representation of upper airway obstruction, depicted on the volume–time plot.

- With advancing age, FEV_1 declines by approximately 25 mL/year in normal subjects, after the age of 35. In smokers with COPD, the decline in FEV_1 is more rapid at approximately 50 mL/year, but may be far more rapid in some, at around 80–100 mL/year. There are no drugs at the time of writing which are proven to alter the natural history of this decline in patients with COPD.
- There is no proven benefit of population screening to identify asymptomatic individuals with COPD. Case finding of undiagnosed

individuals who are at-risk may be helpful, to identify those who would benefit symptomatically from treatment.

- The value of FEV_1 (expressed as percentage predicted) is one of the strongest predictors of mortality in those with COPD.
- In the Framingham cohort study, VC was a major independent predictor of cardiovascular morbidity and mortality.[14]
- A smoking history of 40+ pack years is the single most predictive finding on history or examination in the diagnosis of airflow obstruction.[15] A presumed diagnosis of COPD in the absence of a smoking history of at least 20 pack years should be questioned, or the possibility of alpha-1 anti-trypsin deficiency considered.
- Patients with large airway obstruction are prone to rapid deterioration. The finding of stridor on examination is an ominous sign and may forewarn of catastrophe. However, stridor is often intermittent, sometimes being postural in severity or provoked by exercise. Apparent improvement of stridor may be misleading.

KEY POINTS

- The FEV_1 is a reflection of airflow and therefore airways function or disease. A reduction of the FEV_1/FVC ratio defines an obstructive defect.
- The severity of an obstructive disease is defined by the FEV_1, expressed as percentage predicted.
- A restrictive process is defined by inability to expand the lungs, which may be caused by disease of lung parenchyma, pleura, respiratory musculature or the chest wall.
- The FVC measures lung volume and a reduction *may* indicate the presence of a restrictive defect.
- Demonstration of a reduction of TLC is required to confirm the presence of a restrictive defect.
- FVC is reduced in around 40% of patients with an obstructive defect, and in these cases usually reflects gas trapping within an expanded RV, rather than a true restrictive process.

4

Airway responsiveness

INTRODUCTION

Airway hyperresponsiveness is the hallmark of asthma. Tests of airway responsiveness are therefore most commonly used to confirm or exclude a diagnosis of asthma. Airway responsiveness is usually gauged by measurement of FEV_1, both before and after pharmacological or physical intervention.

Two types of airway responsiveness testing may be employed. More common is reversibility testing, in which a bronchodilator agent is given in an attempt to reverse existing pathological airflow limitation. Less commonly employed is airway challenge testing, in which a bronchoconstrictor stimulus is administered to elicit the abnormal bronchial hyperresponsiveness which characterises asthma.

Baseline spirometry helps to suggest the appropriate form of airways responsiveness testing. Reversibility testing is of limited value in patients with normal or near-normal pre-test spirometry, since measurable improvement is unlikely. Rather, challenge testing is more appropriate in subjects with normal or near-normal spirometric values. Under these circumstances, challenge testing is a highly sensitive test and particularly useful to help exclude asthma when other clinical and lung function findings are not clear-cut, such that the probability of diagnosis is felt to be 'intermediate'.

KEY POINT

Pharmacological challenge tests have a high degree of sensitivity, so a negative test makes a diagnosis of asthma unlikely.

TEST PHYSIOLOGY

The airway calibre of normal, healthy individuals responds on exposure to an appropriate stimulus. A distinguishing feature of asthmatic airways is hyperresponsiveness, meaning that the bronchoconstrictor response may occur at a far lower threshold than would be seen in a healthy individual.

TEST DESCRIPTIONS

Tests of airway responsiveness tend to be time consuming in comparison to other pulmonary function tests, due to the delay required for a specific intervention to take effect. Good subject compliance with reproducible baseline results is requisite to performing responsiveness testing.

Various pre-test conditions and contraindications for tests of airway responsiveness should also be considered before making a referral for this type of test.[16,17] These are similar to those for simple spirometry, outlined in Chapter 3, but in addition include avoidance of any agent which may influence airway responsiveness or tone such as caffeine or antihistamines.

REVERSIBILITY

Reversibility testing involves the evaluation of airway function before and after the administration of a bronchodilator agent. The agent(s) may be a beta-2 agonist, an anticholinergic, or both in combination.

The bronchodilator may be administered by an inhaler, preferably with a spacer to improve airway deposition, or using a nebuliser. The agent, dose, and method of administration should be recorded, along with any deviation from pre-test criteria and test performance technique, as all of these may influence the final response. There is no consensus as to the best protocol, but the most common employs Salbutamol 400 µg.

An appropriate interval should then be allowed for the chosen bronchodilator to reach its maximum effect. For short-acting beta-2 agonists, a delay of 15–20 minutes is required before post-bronchodilator measurements are made, whereas 45 minutes is required after short-acting anticholinergics.

To ensure the maximal sensitivity of the test, the subject should have received no other bronchodilator in the hours prior to the test according to the duration of action of the drug in question. For example, a short-acting bronchodilator such as Salbutamol should not have been taken for at least 4 hours prior to testing.

CHALLENGE TESTING

Pharmacological challenge tests involve administration of incremental dosages of a bronchoconstrictor substance and assessing changes in airway function after each incremental dose. Commonly used bronchoconstrictor substances include Methacholine and Mannitol. The agents may be administered by various methods, but the most common is by a nebulised dosimeter.

Other challenge tests include exercise and cold air, which involve exposing the patient to the relevant stimuli, followed by interval assessment of airway function.

As with reversibility testing, challenge tests should not be performed if bronchodilator medication has been taken within its duration of effect. Caffeine and antihistamines should also be avoided prior to testing.

There are contraindications to performing challenge testing to avoid the potential for causing respiratory distress due to significant and acute bronchoconstriction. The most common of these is marked pre-existing airflow limitation. A pre-challenge FEV_1 of less than 60% of the patient's predicted value is a relative contraindication to challenge testing, which should only proceed in the presence of a compelling clinical need. An FEV_1 of less than 50% predicted is an absolute contraindication.

Safety precautions are required, should severe airway constriction occur. If a challenge test reveals evidence of bronchoconstriction then a bronchodilator should be administered to restore pre-test airway function. Nebulised bronchodilators, supplemental oxygen, and adrenaline should be readily available in case of a severe reaction, and these tests should only be performed within proximity of an emergency medical response team.

INTERPRETATION OF RESULTS

REVERSIBILITY

Guidelines differ in their recommendations for the threshold of significance of a change in FEV_1 following bronchodilator.

The British Thoracic Society (BTS)/Scottish Intercollegiate Guidelines Network (SIGN) guidelines state that an absolute change in FEV_1 of more than 200 ml and 12% is required to be confident of a positive reversibility test.[4] However, the SIGN guidelines also make the point that variability of FEV_1 by 200ml is not specific to asthma and may also occur in those with COPD. SIGN state that an improvement in FEV_1 of 400ml strongly suggests a diagnosis of asthma, being highly unlikely to occur in those with COPD.

The international Global Initiative for Asthma (GINA) report suggests a change in FEV_1 from baseline of 200 mL and >12% is sufficient to confirm significant variability of airflow limitation, though notes that greater confidence in diagnosis of asthma is given by a change of 400 mL and 15%.[11]

A diagnosis of chronic obstructive pulmonary disease (COPD) should not be made if normal spirometry can be achieved after bronchodilator administration, as such a finding would indicate asthma.

Alternatively, airway function may be assessed by measurement of airway resistance, before and after a bronchodilator (see Chapter 8). Measurement of airway resistance is extremely sensitive to very small changes in airway calibre following bronchodilators and can reveal improvements which may not be observed with measurement of the FEV_1. However, measurement of airway resistance is less reproducible than the FEV_1, and so a change in airway resistance following bronchodilator administration of greater than 40% (body plethysmography) or 20%–25% (oscillometry) is required to be confident of a significant positive response.

Static lung volumes (see Chapter 7), such as inspiratory capacity, functional residual capacity, and residual volume may also show a response to reversibility testing. Indeed, in hyperexpanded patients with COPD these measures may be more sensitive than FEV_1.[18]

> **KEY POINT**
>
> Absence of spirometric improvement after use of inhaled bronchodilator therapy does not exclude the possibility of therapeutic benefit. A beneficial effect upon functional residual capacity (FRC), inspiratory capacity, or other lung volumes effect may be occurring, which is not detected by spirometric measurements alone.

CHALLENGE TESTING

As with reversibility testing, FEV_1 is invariably used to assess results of challenge testing due to its high degree of reproducibility. Most pharmacological challenge tests are evaluated by the dose or concentration of bronchoconstrictor required to produce a 20% reduction in FEV_1. These are known as the PD_{20} (provocative dose) or PC_{20} (provocative concentration), respectively.

To perform the test, a subject is given increasing doses or concentrations of bronchoconstrictor via a nebuliser, up to the protocol maximum (e.g. 16 mg mL^{-1} for Methacholine). The FEV_1 is plotted for each concentration (Figure 4.1). A reduction in FEV_1 of 20% constitutes a positive result for a Methacholine challenge if it occurs at a dose of less than 8 mg mL^{-1} according to the current BTS/SIGN asthma management guidelines.[4] The exact dose at which this occurs is determined by interpolation. An increase in airway resistance of greater than 40% measured using oscillometry also indicates a positive challenge test (see Chapter 8).

Results of Mannitol challenge tests are expressed as PD_{15}, or the dose producing a 15% reduction in FEV_1. A reduction in FEV_1 of greater than 15% following an exercise challenge test is diagnostic of exercise-induced bronchoconstriction.

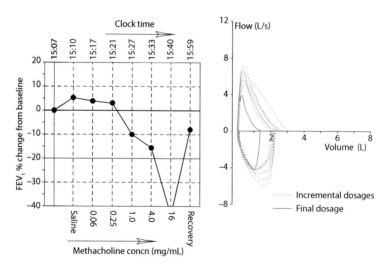

Figure 4.1 A positive Methacholine challenge test. The graph shows changes in FEV_1 in response to various concentrations of Methacholine. A nebulised dose of saline is administered as a control, followed by incremental doses of Methacholine. The reduction in FEV_1 crosses the threshold of 20% between administration of 4.0 and 16 mg/mL. FEV_1 then recovers towards normal after administration of a bronchodilator agent.

The results of challenge testing may also be used to indicate the severity of asthma following a positive response.

Table 4.1 shows levels of severity indicated by pharmacological and exercise challenge results.

Table 4.1 Severity description of response to pharmacological and exercise challenge tests

Asthma severity	Pharmacological challenge PC_{20} (mg mL^{-1})	Exercise challenge maximum drop in FEV_1 (%)
Normal/negative response	>8	<10
Borderline (equivocal response)	4.0–16.0	10–15
Mild	2.0–4.0	15–25
Moderate	0.25–4.0	25–50
Severe	<0.25	>50

KEY POINTS

- Tests of airway responsiveness evaluate lability of airway function.
- Positive responses to reversibility or challenge testing are suggestive of asthma, but not entirely specific.
- A negative challenge test result makes a diagnosis of asthma unlikely.
- COPD is excluded if reversibility testing improves spirometry to within normal values.

5

Fractional concentration of exhaled nitric oxide

INTRODUCTION

Measurement of fractional concentration of exhaled nitric oxide (FE_{NO}) is not strictly a test of respiratory function in the same way as those covered elsewhere in this book, as it does not relate to the structure, mechanics, or physiology of the respiratory system. However, this test is increasingly used and may have a useful role in the management of asthma. The measurement of FE_{NO} is quick, convenient, and non-invasive.

Elevated FE_{NO} levels have been found to correlate with both airway eosinophilia and steroid responsiveness. In this way, an elevated FE_{NO} may support a clinical diagnosis of asthma, though can never exclude asthma as not all asthmatics have airway eosinophilia.

TEST DESCRIPTION/TECHNIQUE

Measurement of FE_{NO} should be made prior to any other pulmonary function tests which require a forced manoeuvre. Such forced manoeuvres may decrease the release of nitric oxide (NO) synthase from the respiratory epithelium, giving a false negative result on subsequent testing.

The test begins with the oral inhalation to a lung volume at or near total lung capacity (TLC). Inhalation through the mouth avoids the possibility of contamination of the sample by NO from the nasal mucosa, which can significantly elevate the result, especially in individuals with rhinitis.

The patient then exhales against a small expiratory pressure in the region of 5 cm H_2O. This small resistance is sufficient to occlude the velum and prevent further contamination of the exhaled sample with nasal NO.

Expiration is performed at a flow of 0.05 Ls^{-1} (±10%) and should continue until a plateau exhaled NO level is reached, at which the level is recorded (see Figure 5.1).[19] This is usually achieved after an expiratory time of >6 seconds,

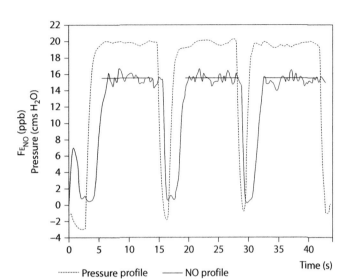

Figure 5.1 Measurement of FE_{NO}. NO concentration (ppb) and airway opening pressure over time showing reproducible profiles and plateaus from the guidelines of the European Respiratory Society (ERS)/American Thoracic Society (ATS). (From American Thoracic S and European Respiratory S, *Am J Respir Crit Care Med*, 171, 912–930, 2005.)

and most measuring equipment requires expiration to continue for about 10 seconds to ensure the presence of an acceptable plateau.

FE_{NO} is often reduced in smokers, making this a very insensitive test for asthma in patients who may smoke as well.

PHYSIOLOGY OF TEST

Patients with asthma cluster into several subtypes, based upon demography, clinical features, and markers of airway inflammation. Although these subtypes are often referred to as phenotypes, there is no strong relationship to specific pathological features. Nonetheless, the categorisation is useful in clinical practice. Increased production of NO is particularly associated with the eosinophilic phenotype. The various phenotypes are summarised in Table 5.1.

NO is produced by NO synthase within airway epithelial cells and has numerous roles, including that of an inflammatory mediator and free

Table 5.1 Asthma phenotypes

Phenotype	Characteristics
Allergic asthma	Typically commences in childhood, associated with atopic disease, responds well to inhaled corticosteroids (ICS). Often eosinophilic.
Non-allergic	Often adults, responds less well to ICS. Neutrophilic, eosinophilic, or scanty airways cellularity (paucigranulocytic).
Late-onset	Often women, non-allergic, may be refractory to ICS.
Fixed airflow	Remodelling of airways may result in fixed and irreversible obstruction after many years of asthma.
Asthma with obesity	Relatively little airway inflammation despite prominent symptoms.

radical with bactericidal properties. Under conditions of disease and increased inflammation, the production of NO is elevated. Increased airway inflammation is a characteristic feature of asthma, particularly when control of symptoms is not optimal. Monitoring of changes in Fe_{NO} levels can provide valuable information regarding the level of inflammation and the effectiveness of therapeutic measures.

NORMAL VALUES AND INTERPRETATION

The current British Thoracic Society guidelines for the management of asthma identify a normal level of Fe_{NO} in adults as being <25 parts per billion (ppb).[4] However, Fe_{NO} levels increase in adulthood and the American Thoracic Society Clinical Practice Guideline takes account of this.[20] Table 5.2 displays recommended Fe_{NO} cut-off values for children and adults.[20]

A Fe_{NO} in the range 20–35 in children or 25–50 in adults is borderline and should be interpreted cautiously with regard to the clinical context.

Following serial measurements, an increase of more than 20% for values over 50 ppb (or >10 ppb for values <50 ppb) should be considered significant and may indicate deteriorating asthmatic control or an impending exacerbation. Similarly, a reduction of Fe_{NO} values of the same magnitude can be considered a significant improvement and represent a positive response to corticosteroid treatment.

Table 5.2 Interpretation of FE_{NO} values in children and adults

FE_{NO} (ppb)		Interpretation	
Children	Adults	Eosinophilic inflammation	Corticosteroid responsiveness
<20	<25	Unlikely	Poor
20–35	25–50	Indeterminate	Indeterminate
>35	>50	Likely	Good

SPECIFIC CONSIDERATIONS

Measurement of FE_{NO} is a relatively new test in respiratory medicine, which has recently made the transition from the research lab to clinical practice. Although its use is strongly supported by some expert opinion, there is as yet little evidence to show better outcomes when management is guided by this tool. In particular, there is insufficient evidence to support withdrawal of inhaled corticosteroids in those without elevation of FE_{NO}.

KEY POINTS

- Elevated FE_{NO} >50 ppb suggests eosinophilic airway inflammation, supporting a diagnosis of asthma.
- In those with a diagnosis of asthma, elevation of FE_{NO} suggests an allergic or eosinophilic phenotype.
- Elevated FE_{NO} >50 ppb suggests steroid responsiveness of airways disease.

6

Gas transfer

INTRODUCTION

Measurement of the lung's ability to transfer gas from the alveoli to the circulation is a fundamental respiratory function test, as it measures directly what the lung really does in life. Gas transfer indices provide a window on the blood–gas barrier and are relatively easy to measure in the lab.

The tracer gas for the measurement of gas transfer is carbon monoxide (CO), used in concentrations below the threshold of toxicity. The very low background concentration of CO, both within the environment and human metabolism, coupled with its high affinity for haemoglobin makes it an ideal tracer substance.

MEASURED INDICES/KEY DEFINITIONS

K_{CO} is the primary measurement which is made of gas transfer. K_{CO} is equivalent to the rate constant of the washout of CO from the lungs, as it equilibrates from the alveoli into the pulmonary capillary blood during the breath-hold phase of the gas transfer test. The K_{CO} represents the average gas-exchange efficiency per unit alveolus or acinus, in units of mmol min^{-1} L^{-1} kPa^{-1}.

TL_{CO} is derived from the product of the K_{CO} and the alveolar volume (V_A):

$$TL_{CO} = K_{CO} \times V_A \qquad (6.1)$$

TL_{CO} is more intuitively understood than K_{CO}, as it represents the performance of the whole system, i.e. both lungs rather than that of a single alveolus. Moreover, it is the more sensitive index of abnormality, making TL_{CO} the preferred index of gas transfer in most situations.

TL_{CO} represents the overall gas diffusing capability of the lung, in SI units of mmol min^{-1} kPa^{-1}. In physics terms, TL_{CO} is the diffusive conductance of the lung to CO. As with other indices, it is expressed in relation to the normal range for age and height. TL_{CO} is a key parameter in the assessment of lung disease.

A NOTE ON NOMENCLATURE

The DL_{CO} (the diffusing capacity of the lung for CO) is synonymous with the TL_{CO} (the transfer factor of the lung for CO). The term DL_{CO} is favoured in the United States, whereas TL_{CO} is favoured in Europe. The term 'capacity' is misleading as it implies that this index represents a maximal value of the lung for gas exchange. However, this is not the case. For example, if the measurement is repeated shortly after exercise, gas transfer increases dramatically in healthy individuals. More accurately, the index represents the diffusing capability of the lung under the standardised protocol used for measurement. Therefore, TL_{CO} is a more accurate and less confusing term, and the one used during the remainder of this text.

ALVEOLAR VOLUME

The alveolar volume (V_A) is the volume of the lungs available for gas exchange, calculated by gas dilution using an inert gas in the test gas mixture. In other words, V_A is the total lung capacity, less any dead space.

Dead space within the lung may be compartmentalised into anatomical and physiological. The anatomical dead space is comprised of the trachea and major airways, which are not involved in gas exchange and total approximately 150 mL. Physiological dead space is an additional component due to poor mixing of inspired gases over the short duration of the time interval (10 seconds) in which V_A is measured. V_A is measured in litres and is reduced by restrictive disease of any cause.

K_{CO}

The K_{CO} is a difficult index for the non-specialist to fully understand and is the subject of much confusion and abuse. The K_{CO} is often misleadingly described as 'the TL_{CO} *corrected* for alveolar volume', due to its arithmetic equivalence with the expression TL_{CO}/V_A. This description is inaccurate in two important ways.

Table 6.1 Primary gas transfer indices

Abbreviation	Units	Name	Comment
V_A	L	Alveolar volume	Lung volume available for gas exchange
K_{CO}	mmol min^{-1} L^{-1} kPa^{-1}	Transfer coefficient	Average gas-exchange efficiency per unit lung volume
TL_{CO}	mmol min^{-1} kPa^{-1}	Transfer factor	Product of TL_{CO} and V_A representing overall performance of lungs for gas exchange

First, K_{CO} is the directly measured parameter, from which the TL_{CO} is derived. Therefore, if either parameter should be considered 'corrected', it is the TL_{CO}.

Second, K_{CO} is not constant as alveolar volume changes. That is to say, a K_{CO} measured at a different alveolar volume would have a different value. The relationship between TL_{CO} and K_{CO} is complex and dependent upon the cause of the lost pulmonary volume[21] (see the section 'Patterns of abnormality').

Table 6.1 summarises the key indices and their meanings.

TEST DESCRIPTION

The measurement of TL_{CO} can be made in several ways, although the single-breath method is now used almost exclusively. The test is simple to perform and can be managed by most subjects, with no contraindications.

Due to the physiological nature of the measurement, adherence to pre-test instructions is important. These include abstinence from smoking, drinking alcohol, eating a large meal, and recent exercise, all of which will produce spurious results. Any other factors which affect metabolism (and blood flow through the lungs) should also be noted and considered during interpretation.

Smoking cigarettes prior to testing administers CO into the circulation, creating a back pressure of CO in pulmonary blood, and thereby increasing the equilibration time constant and reducing the K_{CO}. Counter-intuitively, the use of supplemental oxygen prior to TL_{CO} measurement may also cause a *reduced* TL_{CO}, as the additional oxygen will compete with CO for binding sites on haemoglobin molecules, again reducing the time constant for K_{CO} transfer. Test results should be corrected for haemoglobin, as anaemia or polycythaemia will alter the oxygen carrying capacity of pulmonary blood and influence the K_{CO}.

The single-breath method involves a steady exhalation to residual volume, a quick inspiration to total lung capacity and breath-hold for 10 seconds, followed by a quick expiration back to residual volume. The patient should maintain a good mouthpiece seal during the breath-hold. A minimum vital capacity (VC) of about 1 L (depending on measuring equipment) is required for accurate gas sampling purposes.

PHYSIOLOGY OF GAS EXCHANGE

The physiology of pulmonary gas exchange is governed by Fick's law of passive diffusion, which states that the diffusion of a gas across a permeable membrane is proportional to the area of the membrane and the pressure gradient between the two sides of the membrane, and inversely proportional to the thickness of the barrier and the solubility of the gas in question.

TL_{CO} describes the total diffusing capability of the lung for CO. Physically, it represents the diffusive conductance (ease of diffusion) of CO across the blood–gas barrier. It is a measure of the surface area available for gas transfer (representative of alveolar volume) and the integrity of that surface. As a function of both alveolar volume and diffusion efficiency, it is affected by alterations of either.

NORMAL VALUES

Because there are more physiological variables affecting the measurement of gas transfer than other lung function tests, results are subject to a wider range of normal variability than many other lung function tests. Consequently, it is more robust to express TL_{CO} and K_{CO} in terms of standard residuals, than to express as percentage predicted. A TL_{CO} with a standard residual more negative than −1.64 indicates abnormality. Causes of a reduction in TL_{CO} are shown in Table 6.2.

Table 6.2 Causes of reduced TL_{CO}

Pathophysiological category	Examples
Incomplete pulmonary expansion	Respiratory muscle weakness
	Diffuse pleural thickening
Reduced lung volume	Pneumonectomy, lobectomy
	Atelectasis
Emphysema	Any type
Interstitial lung disease	Idiopathic pulmonary fibrosis
	Sarcoidosis
	Hypersensitivity pneumonitis
	Connective tissue disease-related ILD
	Drug toxicity
Pulmonary vascular disease	Primary pulmonary hypertension
	Pulmonary emboli
Interstitial pulmonary oedema	Heart failure
Artefactual	Anaemia (correction factor should be applied)
	CO back-pressure from smoking

PATTERNS OF ABNORMALITY

Several major patterns of abnormality may be distinguished by the relative changes of the TL_{CO}, K_{CO}, and V_A, determined by the respective losses of volume and function of the gas-exchanging alveoli (see Tables 6.3 and 6.4).

Table 6.3 summarises the patterns of abnormality and relative changes in V_A, K_{CO}, and TL_{CO} for a variety of respiratory disease states. Table 6.4 gives numerical examples, illustrating the different values of K_{CO} which may arise in cases with similar TL_{CO}.

INCOMPLETE LUNG EXPANSION

Lung expansion may be limited in subjects with otherwise normal lungs, for example in patients with weakness of the respiratory musculature or pathological pleural thickening. A similar scenario arises in a normal individual who does not take a maximal inspiration during the gas transfer test.

Table 6.3 Characteristic patterns of change in gas transfer indices in disease

Defect	V_A	K_{CO}	TL_{CO}	Examples
Incomplete expansion	↓	↑↑	↓	Neuromuscular disease
Discrete loss of units	↓	↑	↓	Lobectomy
Diffuse loss of units	↓	↓	↓↓	Idiopathic pulmonary fibrosis
Pulmonary emphysema	↔	↓	↓	Pulmonary emphysema
Pulmonary vascular disorders	↔	↓	↓	Pulmonary arterial hypertension
Increased pulmonary perfusion	↔	↑	↑	Left to right cardiac shunt
Alveolar haemorrhage	↓	↑	↑	Goodpasture's syndrome

Table 6.4 Relationship between TL_{CO}, K_{CO}, and V_A in various lung pathologies

Diagnosis	TL_{CO} (%)	K_{CO} (%)	V_A (%)	Comment
Muscle weakness	59	130	50	Incomplete lung expansion
Pneumonectomy	58	111	51	Discrete loss of units
Diffuse ILD	54	84	66	Diffuse loss of units
Pulmonary emphysema	54	59	91	Alveolar capillary damage/destruction
Idiopathic pulmonary hypertension	56	58	96	Microvascular damage

Source: Reprinted from Hughes JM and Pride NB, *Am J Respir Crit Care Med*, 186, 132–139, 2012. With permission from the American Thoracic Society.

Incomplete expansion reduces the V_A component of the TL_{CO} equation. Consequently, the alveolar surface area to volume ratio of the lungs is *increased*, so that the gas-exchanging efficiency of those alveoli which are open is improved. Therefore, the K_{CO} is increased. Under conditions of incomplete pulmonary expansion, in which the lungs are otherwise normal, the K_{CO} may lie in the range 120%–150% predicted. Nonetheless, the elevation of K_{CO} is proportionately less than the reduction in V_A, making for an overall *reduction* in TL_{CO}.

DISCRETE LOSS OF LUNG UNITS

This situation only arises in its pure form following pulmonary resection surgery, such as a lobectomy or pneumonectomy, in a subject whose remaining lung parenchyma is healthy. Under these circumstances, alveolar volume is predictably reduced. Therefore, the cardiac output is directed through a smaller pulmonary circulation, increasing perfusion of the remaining parenchyma and consequently the K_{CO}. Under such conditions of 'discrete loss of units', the K_{CO} achieves lesser elevation than may be seen under conditions of incomplete expansion and may lie in the range 100%–120%. Therefore, the TL_{CO} is reduced to a lower value than under conditions of incomplete expansion of the lung.

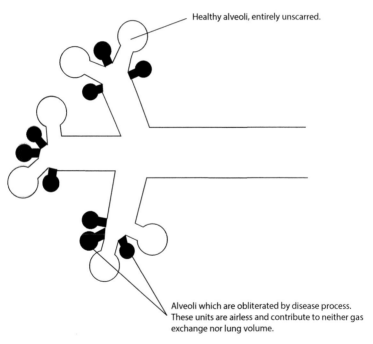

Healthy alveoli, entirely unscarred.

Alveoli which are obliterated by disease process. These units are airless and contribute to neither gas exchange nor lung volume.

Figure 6.1 Discrete loss of units. The effect of disease is limited to a proportion of alveoli, sparing others. Those units which are affected are entirely obliterated, limiting the alveolar volume to healthy units. The overall effect is a loss of volume.

Pulmonary resection is the only perfect model in which completely normal lung remains, despite loss of volume. However, a 'discrete loss of units' scenario may also arise if pulmonary pathology destroys some alveoli entirely, leaving others completely unscathed. This may occur in the presence of localised areas of fibrosis, granulomatous infiltration, or early interstitial lung disease (ILD). Figure 6.1 illustrates such a pattern of disease.

Under these circumstances of very focal disease, inhaled air is directed only to alveoli in which function is intact. The effect is equivalent to a loss of volume, leaving normal function in that volume which remains. This leaves TL_{CO} reduced in similar proportion to V_A, with relative preservation of K_{CO}, which may be normal or even somewhat greater than predicted.

DIFFUSE LOSS OF LUNG UNITS

ILD, such as idiopathic pulmonary fibrosis (IPF), may progress to cause a diffuse loss of lung units throughout the lungs, in which all alveoli are damaged somewhat. In this scenario, inhaled air is directed to alveoli which do not function completely. Destruction of pulmonary vasculature and thickening of the alveolar–capillary membrane reduce gas-exchange efficiency and consequently K_{CO} (Figure 6.2).

Furthermore, the fibrotic process causes increased stiffness of the lungs, with loss of volume in a restrictive process. Therefore, volume is reduced in addition to K_{CO}. TL_{CO} is consequently reduced by both its constituent elements (K_{CO} and V_A), causing a compounded reduction in overall gas-exchange capability.

The relative changes in K_{CO} and TL_{CO} depend on the nature, stage, and progress of the disease. Many patients with early ILD present with a TL_{CO} around 60% predicted and K_{CO} of around 80% predicted.

PULMONARY EMPHYSEMA

Pulmonary emphysema leads to destruction of alveolar septae, which reduces the surface area for gas exchange, but not the lung volume (Figure 3.4). Therefore, TL_{CO} is reduced in similar proportion to the K_{CO}.

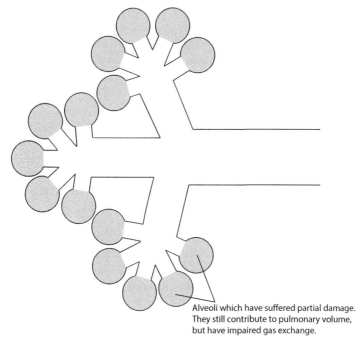

Alveoli which have suffered partial damage.
They still contribute to pulmonary volume,
but have impaired gas exchange.

Figure 6.2 Diffuse loss of units. No alveoli remain unscarred, but they continue to function somewhat. Thus, alveolar volume is relatively maintained, but function is impaired throughout.

KEY POINT

A reduction in TL_{CO} may be caused by either a reduction in V_A (incomplete expansion, discrete loss of units) or a reduction in K_{CO} (emphysema, pulmonary arterial hypertension). Loss of both V_A and K_{CO} occurs in the diffuse loss of units pattern, seen in some cases of ILD, or when ILD coexists with either pulmonary hypertension or emphysema.

PULMONARY VASCULAR DISEASE

The pulmonary vasculopathy seen in pulmonary artery hypertension is associated with thickening of the blood–gas barrier, reducing K_{CO} deleteriously.

Lung volumes are well maintained, in the absence of other coexisting pathology. Consequently, the TL_{CO} is decreased in similar proportion to the K_{CO}. When pulmonary hypertension occurs in isolation from other pulmonary disease, K_{CO} and TL_{CO} may be the only abnormal lung function parameters.

CAUSES OF INCREASED GAS TRANSFER

Increased pulmonary blood volume

Any factor which increases the pulmonary blood volume will make for an increase in K_{CO} and consequently the TL_{CO}. Exercise is a physiological example of this which illustrates the importance of performing the gas transfer measurement under standardised controlled conditions. A left to right cardiac shunt creates a pathological situation where pulmonary blood volume is increased, with a corresponding increase in both K_{CO} and TL_{CO}.

Alveolar haemorrhage

Free blood in the alveoli has a predictable but surprisingly large effect on gas transfer. A small amount of free blood in the alveoli causes a large elevation in K_{CO} due to the free availability of haemoglobin to bind with the CO test gas. V_A may be slightly reduced due to the decrease in compliance associated with extra fluid in the lungs. Therefore, TL_{CO} will also be increased, but to a slightly lesser extent than the K_{CO}.

Although this interesting finding is often mentioned in textbooks, it has little practical utility. Patients presenting with significant pulmonary haemorrhage are usually extremely unwell and hypoxic, so that pulmonary function testing is not clinically appropriate.

Asthma

Both K_{CO} and TL_{CO} may be increased in patients with asthma.

Obesity

K_{CO} may be increased in obese subjects.

CLINICAL PEARLS

INTERSTITIAL LUNG DISEASE

- TL_{CO} is the most sensitive test of lung function for detection of early ILD.
- When severe emphysema coexists with ILD, both FEV_1 and forced vital

capacity (FVC) may be paradoxically well preserved. The increased stiffness of the lung parenchyma which occurs in fibrotic lung disease tends to hold open airways in expiration, facilitating lung emptying.

- Adaptive mechanisms appear to compensate for the decline in gas transfer in the early stages of ILD. Therefore, breathlessness is not usually a feature in patients with early ILD until the TL_{CO} has fallen to a value in the region of 60% predicted. The corollary is that a TL_{CO} within the normal range virtually excludes ILD as a cause of gradual-onset dyspnoea. Occasionally, subjects may notice impairment when TL_{CO} remains relatively well preserved, particularly if gifted with a pre-morbid gas transfer at the upper end of the normal range, e.g. 120% predicted.
- The K_{CO} is better preserved in patients with pulmonary fibrosis than those with emphysema, for the equivalent level of impairment of TL_{CO}.
- Therefore, if K_{CO} is also deleteriously impaired in a patient with ILD (approaching the value of V_A), then the presence of coexisting disease, such as emphysema or pulmonary hypertension, is suggested.
- Occasionally, K_{CO} may be normal in patients with ILD, or even greater than predicted if measured early in the course of their disease. Thus, TL_{CO} is the more sensitive measure of abnormality in this setting.
- TL_{CO} is the single lung function test which best predicts mortality in patients with ILD. However, for charting deterioration over a period of time, FVC is the more reproducible measure. Most major trials of treatment for IPF use interval change of FVC as the primary outcome measure.
- Deterioration in two sequential measurements of TL_{CO} is probably significant if the absolute value has dropped by 15% from baseline. Greater significance may be ascribed to a smaller change in TL_{CO}, if corroboration is provided by deterioration of other parameters, e.g. FVC, radiological, or functional deterioration.

OBSTRUCTIVE DISEASE

- TL_{CO} remains well preserved in patients with obliterative bronchiolitis, until the FEV_1 falls below 1 L or so. This is by contrast to chronic obstructive pulmonary disease (COPD), in which TL_{CO} falls at an early stage, due to the loss of alveolar septae.
- TL_{CO} may be useful in discriminating between asthma and COPD, with the latter causing deleterious reduction in TL_{CO}, which is well preserved

in patients with asthma. This test is not required routinely, but may be helpful in equivocal cases, such as asthmatics with a smoking history, or those with relatively fixed, irreversible airways obstruction.

KEY POINTS/SUMMARY

- TL_{CO} is the product of the alveolar volume (V_A) and the transfer coefficient (K_{CO}).
- K_{CO} is *not* the TL_{CO} corrected for lung volume, as the K_{CO} is the primary physiological measurement, not the TL_{CO}.
- TL_{CO} is reduced by any condition which reduces volume, gas-exchange efficiency, or both.
- The pattern of change in TL_{CO}, V_A, and K_{CO} may be used to differentiate between underlying pathologies.

ACUTE DISEASE

- Measurement of gas transfer is neither particularly helpful nor practicable in the assessment of patients with acute-onset dyspnoea.
- TL_{CO} may be surprisingly well preserved in subjects with pulmonary embolism (PE), though suspicion of untreated PE is a contraindication to performing the forced manoeuvres required for measurement of spirometry.

7

Static lung volumes and lung volume subdivisions

INTRODUCTION

Dynamic lung volume tests such as spirometry are limited to measurement of volumes of gas which may be inspired or expired from the lungs. However, a residual volume (RV) of gas remains within the lungs, even at full expiration. Measurement of this volume provides additional information to supplement the spirometric values, see Figure 7.1.

Lung volumes which cannot be measured by spirometry alone are termed *static* lung volumes. Measurement of static lung volumes may be helpful to evaluate the cause of a reduced forced vital capacity (FVC), particularly if there is suspicion of a mixed restrictive/obstructive defect.

Static volumes are measured less often than gas transfer and may not always be performed in a routine lab assessment, unless requested for a specific indication.

MEASURED INDICES/KEY DEFINITIONS

Measurement of functional residual capacity (FRC) also allows calculation of lung volume subdivisions and derived parameters. Figure 7.1 shows a spirometry trace with all lung volume subdivisions. The major indices calculated during the measurement of static lung volumes are shown in Table 7.1.

The total lung capacity (TLC) is the sum of the vital capacity (VC) and the RV, so TLC = RV + VC.

The RV is often expressed as the proportion of TLC, thus RV/TLC. This ratio represents the proportion of the lungs which is not available for ventilation (but does participate in gas exchange). As such, it is an indirect index of gas trapping.

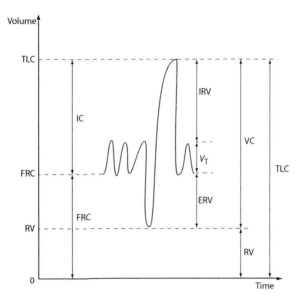

Figure 7.1 Spirometry showing lung volume subdivisions. Note that spirometry cannot measure residual volume, nor any lung volume subdivisions of which residual volume is a component. TLC, total lung capacity; FRC, functional residual capacity; RV, residual volume; IRV, inspiratory reserve volume; V_T, tidal volume; ERV, expiratory reserve volume; VC, vital capacity; IC, inspiratory capacity.

Table 7.1 The principle lung volume subdivisions

Abbreviation	Parameter	Description
RV	Residual volume	The volume of gas remaining in the lungs at the end of a maximal expiration.
TLC	Total lung capacity	The total volume of gas in the lungs at full inspiration.
FRC	Functional residual capacity	The volume of gas remaining in the lungs at the end of a normal resting tidal expiration.
ERV	Expiratory reserve volume	The volume of gas which can be expired from end tidal expiration (FRC) to residual volume.
IC	Inspiratory capacity	This is the volume of gas which can be inspired from FRC to TLC.

TEST DESCRIPTIONS/TECHNIQUES

A variety of methods exist for measurement of static lung volumes, each of which requires differing levels of comprehension, cooperation, and compliance to produce accurate and meaningful results. The three main techniques for measuring static lung volumes are helium dilution, nitrogen washout, and whole-body plethysmography.

HELIUM DILUTION

Helium dilution is the easiest method to perform, but is not the cheapest due to the relative expense of helium gas. There are no contraindications, and the only real pre-requisite is the ability to maintain an effective mouthpiece seal. Some patients will find breathing from a mouthpiece for an extended period of time unpleasant which may influence their normal tidal breathing.

The test begins with a period of normal tidal breathing to establish a consistent end-expiratory volume (FRC), at which point the patient is connected to a closed circuit containing the test gas (Figure 7.2). This gas contains a known concentration of helium, along with sufficient oxygen for the test duration, with the balance made up of nitrogen. The breathing circuit also contains a carbon dioxide absorber such as soda lime to prevent the accumulation of carbon dioxide. Tidal breathing continues until the concentration of helium in the breathing circuit stabilises, indicating equilibration between lungs and the circuit, and relatively thorough mixing and even distribution throughout the lungs. The patient then performs a VC manoeuvre (full inspiration followed by full expiration, or vice versa) to complete the measurement.

At the point where the patient is switched into the breathing circuit (assumed to be at FRC), certain values are known:

V_1 is the volume of the breathing circuit and bag.

C_1 is the concentration of helium in the breathing circuit and bag.

V_2 is the (unknown) volume of gas within the lungs at the beginning of the test (FRC).

The concentration of helium in the lungs is 0%.

At the end of the measurement, V_1 is unchanged, but C_1 will be reduced by dilution with the gas in the lungs which contained no helium.

C_2 is the final concentration of helium within the breathing circuit, measured at the end of the test.

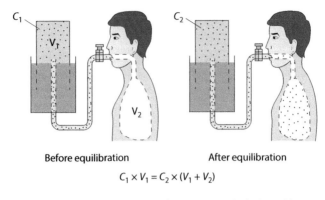

Before equilibration   **After equilibration**

$$C_1 \times V_1 = C_2 \times (V_1 + V_2)$$

Figure 7.2 Method of measuring total lung capacity by helium dilution.

The total gas volume in the lungs and the bag combined is given by $V_1 + V_2$. As the breathing circuit is closed and no helium is added or lost:

$$C_1 \times V_1 = C_2 \times (V_1 + V_2)$$

Rearranging:

$$V_2 = \frac{V_1(C_1 - C_2)}{C_2}$$

As the measurement was commenced with the patient at FRC, V_2 gives a measurement of FRC.

Once the volume of FRC is known, it is easy to calculate the remaining lung volume subdivisions, thus:

$$RV = FRC - ERV$$

$$TLC = RV + VC$$

Alternatively, TLC can be calculated by adding FRC to inspiratory capacity (IC), measured from spirometry.

NITROGEN WASHOUT

Like helium dilution, this technique involves breathing from a closed circuit for a period of time and then performing a VC manoeuvre to provide values for IC, expiratory reserve volume (ERV), and VC. There is no difference in the measurement procedure from the point of view of the patient.

The principle of measurement differs slightly, using nitrogen rather than helium as the test gas. The methods differ in that the tracer gas (nitrogen) exists in the lungs whereas helium does not.

At the point where the patient is switched into the closed circuit (again at FRC), only the concentration of nitrogen within the lungs is known (80%), and this becomes C_L. From this point, the patient breathes 100% oxygen, which continues long enough to 'wash out' the vast majority of nitrogen from the lungs (usually 7 minutes). At the end of the test, the total volume of expired gas is measured, which becomes V_E. The concentration of nitrogen in this expired gas is also measured and becomes C_E. Measurement of FRC, which in this case becomes V_{FRC}, is then easily derived using the following equation:

$$V_{FRC} \times C_L = V_E \times C_E$$

Rearranging:

$$V_{FRC} = \frac{V_E \times C_E}{C_L}$$

Once this value is obtained, then calculation of other lung volume subdivisions is made as for helium dilution.

WHOLE-BODY PLETHYSMOGRAPHY

Measurement is made in a closed whole-body plethysmograph or body box for short (Figure 7.3). This method is generally considered the gold standard, though those who suffer with claustrophobia may be unable to tolerate the procedure. The apparatus required is more bulky (and expensive) than that required for dilution methods. The principle of measurement depends upon Boyle's law, which states that in a closed container, the pressure of a fixed mass of gas is inversely proportional to the volume. In other words, if volume halves, pressure doubles.

The test procedure starts with the patient breathing normally in and out through a standard mouthpiece. Once a consistent breathing pattern and

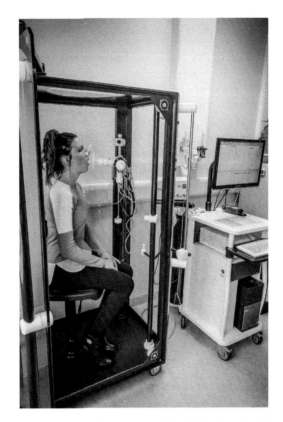

Figure 7.3 Whole-body plethysmograph (or body box for short). (Courtesy of P Pearson and D Gore.)

end-expiratory volume have been established, a shutter is closed at end expiration, following which the patient makes several panting efforts in and out against the shutter. These efforts expand and compress the gas in the lungs according to Boyle's law. The shutter is then released, allowing the patient to take a maximal inspiration to TLC.

The equation required to calculate FRC is slightly more complicated than the dilution or washout techniques, but the principle is similar. At the start of the measurement, the box volume and pressure and alveolar pressure (which with an open glottis is the same as that measured at the mouth) are known. Using these known parameters, the volume of gas in the lung can be calculated from changes in box volume and pressure and mouth pressure during closed-shutter panting.

COMPARISON OF METHODS

Each of these methods employs a different concept and consequently measures a slightly different physical volume. Washout and dilution techniques measure only that gas in the alveoli and airways which is in communication with the breathing circuit. In severe obstructive diseases, gas trapped in closed airways mixes poorly with that in the circuit. Consequently, helium dilution and nitrogen washout may underestimate static lung volumes in subjects with obstructive airways disease.

By contrast, whole-body plethysmography measures all the gas present within the thoracic cavity which is subject to the pressure changes of the closed-shutter panting manoeuvre. This includes any gas trapped behind closed airways and bullae (Figure 7.4), but may also include intestinal gas. This leads to an overestimate of TLC, although error is not usually large. In those with severe obstruction, changes in lung compliance may also

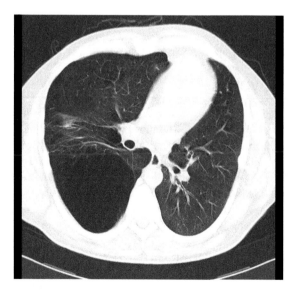

Figure 7.4 Computed tomography (CT) of an emphysematous bulla. The volume of this bulla would not be included in the volume of TLC measured by a dilution method, which would underestimate the true TLC.

interfere with accurate pressure transmission from the lungs to the mouth during the panting manoeuvre. Nonetheless, measurement of static lung volumes by whole-body plethysmography in obstructive airways disease is more accurate than that measured by gas dilution or washout techniques.

The difference between TLC measured by dilution or washout, and that measured by whole-body plethysmography provides a useful additional index of the extent of any gas trapping in obstructive airway disease.

The only situation where dilution or washout techniques may be preferable to whole-body plethysmography is where the patient is unable to manage this technique due to claustrophobia, habitus, or disability.

PHYSIOLOGY OF LUNG VOLUMES

TOTAL LUNG CAPACITY

During inspiration, the chest wall musculature expands the lungs against the force of their elastic recoil, which would otherwise tend to deflate them, like a balloon. As the lungs expand they become progressively stiffer, i.e. their compliance is reduced. The lungs reach TLC when the force generated by the inspiratory respiratory muscles is no longer able to overcome the force generated by the elastic recoil of the lungs and chest wall.

RESIDUAL VOLUME

In young healthy subjects, expiration can progress no further when the ribs are opposed, so that the RV is determined by the anatomical mechanics of the chest wall. This typically occurs at an RV of approximately 25% of TLC.

However, with increasing age, airway closure occurs during deep expiration, resulting in gas trapping at progressively higher RVs, and thereby forms the limiting factor to expiration. Typically, RV may occur at up to 40% of TLC in the elderly. As such, the RV is one of the few lung volumes that increase with age. This gas trapping may be increased markedly in those with emphysema.

FUNCTIONAL RESIDUAL CAPACITY

This is the volume within the lungs at the end of a passive expiration. Expiration during normal tidal breathing is a passive manoeuvre, achieved by relaxation of the respiratory musculature against an open glottis. FRC occurs at the point at which outward recoil of the chest wall balances the inward recoil of the lungs.

Therefore, FRC reflects the compliance of the lungs and chest wall, both of which may be affected by disease. The FRC will also be reduced when a subject moves from an upright to a supine posture, as the abdominal contents push against the diaphragm in the supine position (particularly in the obese).

The FRC is an important concept, as it provides a reservoir which maintains blood oxygenation during any pause in breathing or apnoea.

CLOSING CAPACITY

Closing capacity is a volume which is not routinely measured by pulmonary function testing, but is important conceptually. Closing capacity is the lung volume at which airway closure begins to occur during expiration. It is physiologically significant because closure of airway units causes them to become unventilated, the consequence of which is ventilation–perfusion mismatch and a reduction in arterial oxygen tension.

Notably, the closing capacity increases with age. By the age of 75 years in a healthy individual, the closing capacity exceeds the FRC in the upright position, meaning that some airway closure occurs all of the time. This is one of the principle reasons for the gradual decrease in arterial oxygen tension seen with ageing. Closing capacity is more likely to exceed FRC in the supine position, in which FRC is lower (though closing capacity unchanged).

NORMAL VALUES

Static lung volume indices are compared to predicted values or standard residuals in a similar way to the majority of lung function test results. Likewise, the relationships between some lung volume subdivisions change predictably with age and in disease.

The predicted TLC varies directly with height, but is greater in men than women of the same height. A TLC of less than 80% of predicted or with a standard residual more than 1.64 below the mean is considered abnormal (see Chapter 1).

The RV is also compared with predicted norms. For example in the average male (1.78 m, 70 kg), with a TLC of around 7 L, RV should lie in the range 1.5–2 L.

The RV is commonly expressed as the proportion of TLC which it occupies, i.e. RV/TLC. This value changes naturally with age, rising from 20%–25% in youth to approximately 40% by the age of 70.

Multiple factors affect the normal value of FRC, including posture, body weight, and gender. Generally though, FRC occurs at about 50% of TLC, but also increases with age (see above). In the supine position, the force of the abdominal viscera against the diaphragm reduces the FRC by approximately 25%.

PATTERNS OF ABNORMALITY

Figure 7.5 shows the pattern of lung volume subdivisions seen in various different disease states.[22]

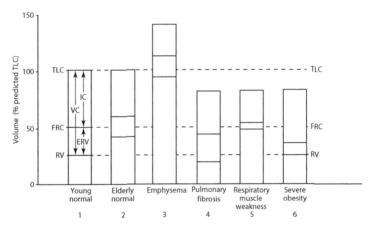

Figure 7.5 Typical changes in lung volume subdivisions by disease. Volume expressed as percent predicted TLC. Horizontal lines indicate FRC. (2) With ageing RV and FRC both increase, so that VC falls within the same TLC. (3) In emphysema the TLC increases, with greater proportional increases in RV and FRC making for a reduction in FVC. (4) In intrapulmonary restriction RV tends to fall or remain unchanged, whereas in muscle weakness (5) RV tends to increase. (6) In obesity, an increase in ERV is characteristic. (Modified from Gibson G, In J Hughes, N Pride [eds.], *Lung Function Tests: Physiological Principles and Clinical Applications*, London, WB Saunders, 1999.)

Relationship between VC and TLC

Reduction of TLC is the defining feature of a restrictive defect (see Table 3.4 for a list of causes). The relative change of other lung volume subdivisions provides additional information, which may indicate the cause of the reduction in TLC.

A reduced TLC is usually associated with a reduction in VC, from which its presence may be suspected by spirometry. However, a reduction in VC is not always associated with a reduced TLC. In up to 50% of cases in which a reduced VC is detected by spirometry, the TLC is normal.[12,23] The reduction of VC in such cases is caused by an increase in the RV, within the same envelope of TLC (see Figure 7.1).

An obstructive defect may frequently be associated with a reduction of VC, due to trapping of gas in small airways thereby increasing the RV. Under these circumstances, the TLC measured by whole-body plethysmography will be normal or even increased.

Conversely, VC may be maintained despite a reduction in TLC, if the RV is reduced. This may occur early in the course of interstitial lung disease (ILD), though it is rare.

Obstructive lung disease

Emphysema causes the greatest elevations of RV seen, due to gas trapping, which prevents complete expiration. During the early course of obstructive airways disease, the RV increases at the expense of FVC, without any increase in TLC (gas trapping). Later in the course of disease, TLC also rises (hyperexpansion).

The FRC is also elevated in obstructive airway disease (hyperinflation) as the greater compliance of emphysematous lungs makes for a reduction of recoil, shifting the lung volume at which inward and outward recoil pressures equilibrate.

Interstitial lung disease

The RV is usually relatively unaffected by ILD, or only reduced in proportion to TLC, so that the RV/TLC remains approximately normal, or only slightly elevated.

The FRC is reduced by ILD, though proportionately less than other lung volume subdivisions.

MISCELLANEOUS

Obesity causes loss of FRC, leading to loss of ERV. Therefore, tidal breathing occurs at smaller FRCs.

The RV is increased in patients with expiratory muscle weakness, due to the reduced force that can be developed to expel air from the lungs. Likewise, the RV/TLC is also increased.

In left ventricular insufficiency, the RV is also increased because pulmonary congestion reduces the compressibility of lung tissue.

Table 7.2 summarises the key changes in static lung volume and lung volume subdivision indices.

SPECIFIC CONSIDERATIONS

ANAESTHESIA

Induction of anaesthesia brings about a further reduction of FRC to 15%–20% below that which occurs in a supine subject. The reduction is seen whether neuromuscular blockade is used or not, and occurs with all anaesthetic drugs. Thus, anaesthesia reduces the FRC to around the level of the closing capacity, which has practical considerations for maintaining oxygenation in the anaesthetised patient.

FRC IN PATIENTS RECEIVING VENTILATORY SUPPORT: PEEP AND CPAP

Mechanical ventilatory support works by providing positive airway pressure to inflate the lung. This is by contrast to spontaneous ventilation, during which the respiratory muscles inflate the lungs by transmission of *negative* pressure from the pleura to the airways. Expiration, under both conditions of spontaneous and mechanical ventilation, is effected passively by the recoil

Table 7.2 Characteristic changes in lung subdivisions in lung disease

Defect	TLC	RV	RV/TLC
Obstructive	↑	↑	↑
Restrictive – ILD	↓	↔/↓	↔/↑
Restrictive – muscle weakness	↓	↑	↑

of the lungs and chest wall, which generates positive airway pressure and thereby outward airflow. Therefore, the patient undergoing mechanical ventilation experiences positive airway pressure throughout the respiratory cycle.

Positive end-expiratory pressure (PEEP) is routinely applied to patients with acute respiratory failure who are undergoing mechanical ventilation. PEEP is a small pressure applied to the airway during expiration, against which a patient must breathe to exhale. This has the favourable effect of increasing FRC. A higher inspiratory pressure is then utilised to elevate the inspiratory volume by the same amount as the increase in FRC, maintaining an equivalent tidal volume.

A similar technique may be employed in the care of spontaneously breathing patients who require respiratory support. Continuous positive airway pressure (CPAP) applies additional positive pressure throughout the respiratory cycle and may be administered through a face mask. Inspiration, under these circumstances is driven by negative pleural pressure but augmented by the additional positive airway pressure. CPAP therefore aids inspiration, whilst providing a resistance to expiration which increases FRC.

The effect of both PEEP and CPAP is to increase FRC. In patients with respiratory failure, this has several advantages:

1. The increase in FRC relative to closing capacity increases the amount of lung that is ventilated throughout the respiratory cycle, thus improving ventilation–perfusion matching and oxygenation (see section 'Closing capacity').
2. Consolidated lung segments tend to collapse at low volumes and the elevation of FRC recruits such segments into participation in ventilation and arterial oxygenation.
3. In patients with pulmonary oedema, the increased volume of ventilated lung increases the capacity of the pulmonary interstitium for water and helps to reduce the volume of alveolar oedema.
4. In patients with stiff and poorly compliant lungs, the increase in FRC shifts the lung to a more favourable point on the pressure–volume compliance curve, so that less work of breathing is required to produce equivalent ventilation.
5. Face-mask CPAP is also used to treat obstructive sleep apnoea (OSA, Figure 7.6). In patients with OSA, the pharynx collapses during sleep, under the negative pressure of inspiration. By maintaining positive airway pressure throughout the respiratory cycle, the upper airway is splinted open during inspiration.

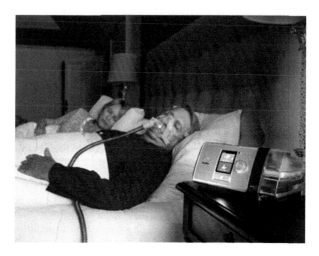

Figure 7.6 Continuous positive airway pressure treatment for obstructive sleep apnoea. (Courtesy of Resmed Limited.)

CLINICAL PEARLS

- In many cases where the FVC is reduced, measurement of TLC does not demonstrate a restrictive defect. Reduction of FVC may otherwise occur in obstructive airways disease, when gas trapping increases the RV, at the expense of FVC. A reduction in FVC may be seen in 40% of chronic obstructive pulmonary disease (COPD) cases. In a large series of reported pulmonary function tests, a reduction in TLC was confirmed in only 10% of those with a reduced FVC, an increased RV accounting for the reduced FVC in the other 90% of cases.[12]
- Measurement of static lung volumes may be useful for evaluating more complex mixed defects, but in order of importance probably comes after spirometry, the flow–volume loop and gas transfer.
- Measurement of lung volumes is requisite to assessment for lung volume reduction surgery, which may occasionally be helpful for patients with severe emphysema, as hyperexpansion (increased TLC) and gas trapping (increased RV) are amongst the criteria.
- There is little role for performing serial measurement of static lung volumes over a period of time to track the course of a subject's condition, neither in obstructive nor ILD. Once the distribution of static

volumes has been determined, any deterioration is likely to correlate with the decline in the values of dynamic lung volumes, measureable by spirometry.

- If a subject has normal spirometry and normal gas transfer, then these findings provide a robust diagnosis of normality. Little would be gained in most situations by measuring static volumes as a further screening measure.

- The IC/TLC ratio may provide a useful index of severity of COPD, as it provides a measure of hyperinflation. This ratio has proven more predictive of mortality than FEV_1 in at least one study of patients with COPD.[24] IC also correlates with exercise tolerance in patients with COPD.

- Many patients with airways disease make a positive volume response to bronchodilator, even if there is no measureable increase in FEV_1. Such a response may be evidenced by an increase in IC whilst RV, TLC and FRC may reduce toward their normal values, measureable only by recording static lung volumes.[18] Moreover, this increase may correlate with an improvement in symptomology. Therefore, lack of response of FEV_1 to bronchodilator does not preclude benefit.

- When a restrictive defect is caused by muscle weakness, the RV is often increased, by contrast to ILD, where the RV is usually either unchanged or slightly reduced.

- The volume which is most susceptible to change in patients with obesity is the ERV, which may be dramatically reduced. A reduction in TLC and VC may also be seen, but is usually limited to around 10%.

KEY POINTS

- Tests of static lung volumes measure indices which cannot be accessed by simple spirometry alone.
- A reduction of TLC is the defining feature of a restrictive defect.
- Many subjects with a reduced FVC do not have a reduction of TLC, i.e. they do not truly have a restrictive defect.
- In patients with obstructive airway disease, gas dilution and washout measurements commonly underestimate TLC compared with whole-body plethysmography.

8

Airway resistance

INTRODUCTION

Airway resistance is the hindrance posed to airflow by the friction between the air itself and the respiratory mucosa. Airway resistance is a key factor in determining airflow, and so may be inferred from the FEV_1 ratio. However, it is sometimes helpful to make direct measurements of airway resistance. Airway resistance is an extremely sensitive index and may detect subtle airway changes below the threshold of detection by spirometric measurements. Moreover, the measurement is truly independent of effort, which may be helpful if there is doubt about volition.

Airway resistance measurements are made routinely in many pulmonary function laboratories, and familiarisation with the measurement indices and their meaning will afford an increased understanding of airway function, mechanics, and characteristics. Nonetheless, airway resistance is a slightly more specialised test than those described in earlier chapters and its usage is more applicable to the respiratory specialist.

Several methods are available for making measurements of airway resistance and related indices including: the pleural pressure method, the interrupter method, whole-body plethysmography, and oscillometry. With the exception of the pleural pressure method, which requires insertion of an oesophageal balloon catheter, the procedures are non-invasive and the technique to produce representative results is manageable by most. All of the methods entail either tidal breathing or gentle panting whilst measurements are made.

The most common method used for measuring airway resistance is the whole-body plethysmography technique due to the wider availability of plethysmographic equipment. However, measurements of airway resistance using oscillometry techniques are rapidly gaining popularity. For this reason, the remainder of this chapter focuses on body plethysmography and oscillometry techniques.

PHYSIOLOGY OF AIRWAY RESISTANCE TESTS

The total impedance to airflow comprises an elastic component due to recoil of the lung parenchyma and chest wall, and a resistive component originating from friction between flowing gas and the airway wall. The latter of these is quantified in the measurement of airway resistance.

The natural tendency of the lung would be to empty like a balloon, if removed from the thorax and thereby uncoupled from the constraints of the chest wall. This is seen in a patient with a pneumothorax, in which the presence of air within the pleural space uncouples the lung in such a way.

On the other hand, the natural tendency of the isolated chest wall would be to spring outward to occupy a larger volume, if uncoupled from the restraining influence of the lungs.

Under conditions of resting tidal breathing, the differing natural relaxation volumes of these two components of the respiratory system makes for a negative pleural pressure throughout the respiratory cycle, as this space exists under the opposing tensions of the lung (tending to empty) and the ribcage (tending to spring outward). (See 'Functional residual capacity' in Chapter 7.)

By contrast, the muscular tension developed in a *forced* expiration generates a positive intrapleural pressure to drive gas outward through the airways. Therefore, during a forced exhalation from total lung capacity (TLC), two forces are active in expelling gas from the lungs:

1. The elastic recoil of the respiratory system, seeking to return the lung to functional residual capacity (FRC).
2. Positive intrapleural pressure generated by the respiratory muscles.

However, as the thoracic cage squeezes alveoli, forcing gas out, it also compresses airways. This creates a tendency for airway collapse, particularly in late expiration. Therefore, the same intrapleural pressure that is *driving* expiration is also *obstructing* it, so that the forces tend to cancel out. This is the principle of the flow-limited portion of the flow–volume curve discussed in Chapter 3. Thus, the elastic recoil of the tissue in which the airways are embedded is the determining factor in maintaining their patency (see Figures 3.2 and 3.3).

Therefore, FEV_1 is determined principally by the parenchymal properties of the lung, rather than the amount of effort applied, making it reproducible. By contrast, peak flow occurs early in expiration, before airway collapse occurs, and is therefore more effort-dependent.

During resting tidal ventilation, the main physiological factors affecting airway resistance are airway tone and lung volume. At smaller lung volumes, the airways are compressed to a smaller diameter, causing a fourth power reciprocal increase in resistance. Airway resistance is therefore a function of the volume at which it is measured. Thus, the specific airway resistance (sR_{aw}) is a useful measure, which standardises airway resistance to the lung volume at which it is measured.

Under conditions of laminar flow, the resistance to gas flow through a rigid tube is described by the Poiseuille equation:

$$\text{Resistance} = \frac{8 \times \text{Tube length} \times \text{Gas viscosity}}{\pi \times \text{Tube radius}^4}$$

However, airflow in the upper airways tends to be turbulent, particularly around airway bifurcations. Under these conditions, resistance to flow is greater than would be predicted by the Poiseuille equation. Resistance to turbulent flow is proportional to the density of the inspired gas and the fifth power of the airway radius. The resistance to turbulent flow is independent of the gas viscosity.

Under all conditions, airflow is driven by the pressure difference between one end of the airway (the mouth) and the other (the alveoli), giving:

$$\text{Flow} = \frac{P_{\text{ALV}} - P_{\text{MOUTH}}}{\text{Resistance}}$$

PLETHYSMOGRAPHY TECHNIQUE

TEST DESCRIPTION/TECHNIQUE

Standardisation of the test technique requires that the patient pant evenly at approximately 60–100 breaths/min (60–100 Hz), achieving a flow of approximately 0.5 L/s. Some patients find this easy, but others will require considerable coaching to achieve the desired breathing pattern.

Multiple traces can be recorded consecutively until consistent results are achieved, with the most representative trace used to report results. However, patients may become uncomfortable if panting continues for too long, as the unnatural breathing pattern may produce transitory symptoms of hyperventilation.

Measured indices/key definitions

The following indices are measured using the body plethysmography technique for assessing airway resistance:

Abbreviation	Parameter	Pronounced	Units
R_{aw}	Airway resistance	Raw	$cmH_2O \, L^{-1} \, s$
G_{aw}	Airway conductance	Gore	$L \, s^{-1} \, cmH_2O^{-1}$
sR_{aw}	Specific airway resistance	S-raw	$cmH_2O \, s$
sG_{aw}	Specific airway conductance	S-gore	$s^{-1} \, cmH_2O^{-1}$

R_{aw} has a hyperbolic relationship to lung volume, rising sharply below FRC. Specific airway resistance is a more standardised index, which is corrected for the lung volume at which the measurement was made, most often FRC.

Airway conductance (G_{aw}) is a measure of how easily air flows through the airways. Conductance is the reciprocal of airway resistance and so has a linear relationship to volume.

The values most commonly reported are R_{aw} and sR_{aw}. Confusion may arise if values for resistance and conductance are reported concurrently, as a high value for one equates to a low value for the other.

Normal values

As with most lung function indices, results are compared with predicted normal values. However, an average airway resistance (R_{aw}) should fall in the range 1–3 $cmH_2O \, L^{-1} \, s$. Values both above and below these suggest pathological change. A normal range for specific airway conductance (sG_{aw}) is 0.13–0.35 $s^{-1} \, cmH_2O^{-1}$.

Patterns of abnormality

Airway resistance is one of the few lung function variables where a value higher than predicted signifies a reduction in functional status. Increases in R_{aw} and sR_{aw} are seen in obstructive airway disease such as asthma and chronic obstructive pulmonary disease (COPD).

More information regarding the nature of increased airway resistance may be obtained from the graphical plot of pressure change against volume throughout the respiratory cycle, which is produced during the airway resistance measurement. Figure 8.1 shows the most commonly encountered graphical displays of airway resistance. The loop described by the test manoeuvre takes on a variety of characteristic shapes in

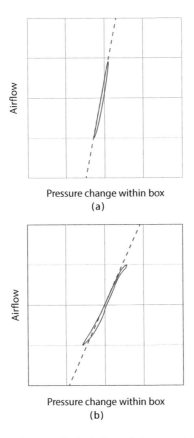

Figure 8.1 Airway resistance. Typical plots of airway resistance – (a) normal, (b) increased expiratory resistance loop in asthma, and (c) large increase in expiratory resistance in COPD. The more oblique the angle of a resistance-trace, the greater the airway resistance.

(*Continued*)

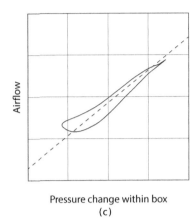

Pressure change within box

(c)

Figure 8.1 (*Continued*) Curve (a) shows a normal pressure–flow relationship, with curves (b) and (c) showing increasingly oblique angles and airway resistance typical in asthma and COPD, respectively.

health and disease. A more complete account of airway resistance tests and abnormal patterns can be found in Ruppel's Manual of Pulmonary Function Testing.[25]

Although interpretation of these can be confusing, essentially the more the loop 'leans over', the greater the airway resistance recording will be. Note that the x-axis represents changes in box pressure, with the y-axis showing changes in flow throughout the panting manoeuvre. The measurement describes how much change in pressure must be developed in order to produce the desired flow. Where airflow limitation exists, more pressure change is required to generate the same flow, producing an oblique curve. The calculated slope of the curve represents the measured airway resistance value.

The next revealing characteristic of the airway resistance loop is the site at which the majority of the flattening of the loop occurs. Flattening at the bottom of the loop suggests high expiratory resistance, as in COPD. Flattening at the top of the loop signifies high end-inspiratory resistance, as seen in variable extrathoracic obstruction (see 'Variable extrathoracic obstruction' in Chapter 3). Flattening at both ends of the airway resistance loop suggests fixed airway obstruction.

OSCILLOMETRY TECHNIQUES

TEST DESCRIPTION/TECHNIQUE

Two methods are available for measuring respiratory impedance by oscillometry. These are the forced oscillometry technique (FOT) and the impulse oscillometry system (IOS). There are technical differences between the two technologies, and a tendency for IOS to feel slightly less comfortable for the patient, but the method for obtaining measurements is identical for both systems.

The test requires that patients perform natural tidal breathing manoeuvres through a mouthpiece for a predetermined period. The period varies amongst different equipment, but is only a matter of seconds. Both FOT and IOS superimpose external pressure/flow signals at multiple frequencies (usually 5–20 Hz) on the natural pattern of spontaneous tidal breathing. These external signals are electronically analysed to determine the relevant impedance parameters of the respiratory tract.

The fact that testing requires only quiet tidal breathing is one of the great advantages of this measuring technique. There are no contraindications, and even individuals who are unable to achieve acceptable spirometry should be capable of producing a reliable assessment of airway function via oscillometry. Reliably performed spirometry is less variable than oscillometry measurements, although oscillometry is more discriminating in peripheral airway obstruction.

Analysis of the various signal frequency spectra can provide additional information on the distribution of increased airway resistance within the bronchial tree. Lower frequency signals (5 Hz) penetrate throughout all airways, whereas higher frequency signals (20 Hz) penetrate only through to the larger central airways. Therefore, isolation of the frequency penetrating to the peripheral airways by subtracting the high-frequency spectrum (5-20 Hz) can provide specific information regarding small airway resistance (see Figure 8.2).

MEASURED INDICES/KEY DEFINITIONS

Table 8.1 describes the indices produced during the measurement of respiratory impedance using oscillometry.

An increase in total airway resistance at 5 Hz (R_5) indicates an increase in overall respiratory resistance. This includes all resistive components of the bronchial tree including extrathoracic, central, and small airways. R_5 alone

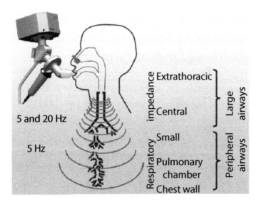

Figure 8.2 Oscillometry with penetration of low- and high-frequency signals through the bronchial tree. (Courtesy of Carefusion Germany Ltd.)

Table 8.1 Key parameters produced during oscillometry measurement

Abbreviation	Parameter	Units
R_5	Resistance (5 Hz)	cm H_2O L^{-1} s or kPa L^{-1} s
R_{20}	Resistance (20 Hz)	cm H_2O L^{-1} s or kPa L^{-1} s
$R_5–R_{20}$	Resistance (5–20 Hz)	cm H_2O L^{-1} s or kPa L^{-1} s
X_5	Reactance (5 Hz)	cm H_2O L^{-1} s or kPa L^{-1} s
Ax	Reactance area	cm H_2O L^{-1} or kPa L^{-1}
F_{res}	Resonant frequency	Hz

cannot identify the distribution of airway resistance, but this can be discerned with reference to the graphical frequency spectra display.

Increases in higher frequency resistance, such as at 20 Hz (R_{20}), suggest increases in central airway or extrathoracic obstruction. Subtraction of R_{20} from R_5 ($R_5–R_{20}$) gives an indication of a specific increase in peripheral airway resistance.

Reactance describes a further element of respiratory impedance. It comprises the inertia of the moving air column (inertance) in the large, central airways, and the elastic properties of lung tissue (capacitance). Reactance tends to be more frequency dependent than resistance. In health, reactance is negative at lower frequencies (the capacitance component) and positive at higher frequencies (the inertance component). Large decreases in low-frequency reactance at 5 Hz (X_5) suggest reduced capacitance due to a loss of tissue elastic recoil such as that seen in emphysema. Changes in the frequency distribution pattern of the reactance spectrum can also suggest the presence of extrathoracic obstruction.

The frequency at which the capacitance and inertance components of the reactance spectrum are equal, i.e. the frequency where reactance crosses zero, is known as the resonant frequency (F_{res}). It represents the frequency at which the total impedance to airflow is exclusively due to airway resistance. F_{res} also increases with the degree of peripheral airways obstruction.

The area of negative reactance between the reactance at 5 Hz (X_5) and the F_{res} is termed the Ax or Goldman triangle, and is a further indication of small airway obstruction and reduced lung elastic recoil.

The usual graphical presentations of healthy resistance and reactance oscillometry spectra traces are shown in Figure 8.3, along with the normal location and appearance of key oscillometry indices.

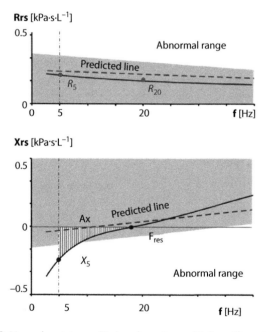

Figure 8.3 Normal resistance (Rrs) and reactance (Xrs) oscillometry spectra showing key oscillometry indices. R_5: Total respiratory resistance measured at 5 Hz, R_{20}: Respiratory resistance measured at 20 Hz, Ax: Area of negative reactance (Goldman triangle), X_5: Reactance at 5 Hz, F_{res}: Resonant frequency. (Courtesy of Carefusion Germany Ltd.)

Normal values

Reference values for airway resistance obtained via oscillometry are less well established than traditional measurements such as spirometry. A selection of reference equation literature is considered in the European Respiratory Society (ERS) Task Force document on the subject for children and adults,[26] although appropriate reference ranges are incorporated within manufacturers' oscillometry system software.

Oscillometry reference values are predominantly height dependent with nearly no age dependence in adults. Therefore, they are less variable than spirometry reference ranges which vary with age.

Patterns of abnormality

Key oscillometry indices change in a characteristic pattern in disease. Typical resistance and reactance frequency spectra are shown in Figures 8.4 and 8.5, respectively.

Increases in central airway resistance, such as those seen in asthma, cause an increase in total airway resistance (R_5). There is little frequency dependence in resistance parameters and minimal change in reactance values. This is shown in curve (b) of Figure 8.4. Values for $R_5 > 140\%$ predicted are considered abnormal.

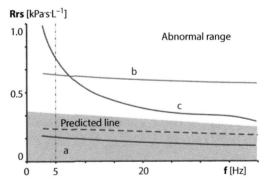

Figure 8.4 Typical resistance oscillometry curves. (a) Normal resistance, (b) central airway obstruction, (c) peripheral obstruction. (Courtesy of Carefusion Germany Ltd.)

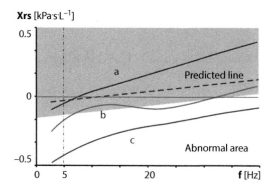

Figure 8.5 Typical reactance frequency spectra curves. (a) Normal reactance, (b) extrathoracic obstruction, (c) peripheral impairment (obstruction/restriction). (Courtesy of Carefusion Germany Ltd.)

Oscillometry performed by patients with emphysema also shows an increase in total resistance (R_5), but with additional frequency dependent increases in resistance at lower frequencies (R_5–R_{20}). Emphysematous changes reduce elastic recoil, increasing peripheral airway resistance. This is displayed on the resistance frequency spectra as an inflection at lower frequencies, with a greater increase in R_5–R_{20} values compared with R_5. Additionally, decreased elastic recoil decreases reactance values, with a more negative X_5 and large increases in both Ax and F_{res}. These changes are represented by curve (c) in Figures 8.3 and 8.4.

Increased small airway resistance in confirmed asthma, indicated by increases in R_5–R_{20} compared with R_{20} with lesser associated changes in X_5, Ax, and F_{res}, may be useful in identifying diminishing asthma control. The Goldman reactance area (Ax) and the resonant frequency (F_{res}) are most useful in the assessment of a bronchodilator response in the small airways. Changes of Ax of 40% and F_{res} of 20% are considered significant.

Deviations in the reactance frequency spectra at higher frequencies may also suggest the presence of extrathoracic airway obstruction. A typical reactance spectrum in extrathoracic airway obstruction is shown in curve (b) in Figure 8.5.

With a supporting clinical history, curve (c) in Figure 8.5 may also suggest the presence of a restrictive defect, although this is less reliable than a reduced vital capacity (VC), and still requires confirmation by lung volume measurement via traditional static lung volume measurement techniques.

In summary, the following general principles can be applied in the interpretation of resistance and reactance oscillometry spectra results.

1. Increased R_5 and little frequency dependence, with normal or minimal changes to the reactance spectra – typical of asthma if R_5 greater than 140% predicted.
2. Increased R_5 but greater increase in R_5–R_{20}, with large changes in X_5, Ax, and F_{res} – typical of emphysema.
3. Increased R_5–R_{20} with slight or no changes in X_5, Ax, and F_{res} – suggests asthma with diminished control.
4. Deviations in higher frequency reactance spectra – suggests extrathoracic obstruction.

ASSESSMENT OF SEVERITY

At present, little literature exists to relate airway resistance to disease severity. However, airway resistances which are in excess of 500% of their predicted value are commonplace in severe COPD.

SPECIFIC AND CLINICAL CONSIDERATIONS

Reversibility: Reversibility is traditionally measured by the change in FEV_1 before and after administration of an appropriate bronchodilator agent. Likewise, reversibility testing may be applied to measurement of airway resistance, providing a more sensitive measure of reversibility, which may not be apparent on spirometry.

Small airways: Measurement of airway resistance may provide greater insight into disease of the small airways, as FEV_1 is governed by dynamic collapse, which is sited within the larger airways. Disease which is localised to these small airways is a feature of some cases of asthma and may respond to treatment with inhaled corticosteroids.

Volition: Importantly, measurement of airway resistance is independent of effort. Therefore, these tests have a role in subjects whose effort is felt to be a limiting factor. These measurements may also be useful to assess airways disease in patients who are unable to perform a forced expiratory manoeuvre, for whatever reason.

One disadvantage of the resistance indices is that they lack the level of repeatability, reliability, and reproducibility of the FEV_1. Therefore, much greater changes in pre- and post-bronchodilator airway resistance values of at least 40% (via body plethysmography) or 20% (via oscillometry) must be achieved to be confident of a significant positive reversibility result.

KEY POINTS/SUMMARY

- The total impedance to airflow comprises an elastic component, due to recoil of the lung parenchyma and chest wall, and a resistive component originating from friction between flowing gas and the airway wall.
- Airway resistance is a fundamental property of the lungs, which determines flow. Resistance is inversely proportional to the fourth power of airway radius, so halving the diameter causes a 16-fold increase in resistance, or greater under conditions of turbulent flow.
- Airway resistance measurements are truly independent of effort, and not subject to a patient's volition.
- Measurements of airway resistance are more sensitive to small airway disease and may provide additional information regarding the degree of airway reversibility.
- Greater use is being made in clinical practice of airway resistance measurements, although they remain the province of the respiratory specialist.

Respiratory muscle strength

9

INTRODUCTION

Tests of respiratory muscle strength are employed when weakness is suspected. Unlike the tests described in previous chapters, they would not be part of routine investigation of breathlessness, unless there was a specific clue to the presence of respiratory muscle weakness, such as orthopnoea or muscle weakness elsewhere. Weakness of the respiratory muscles may be due to disease at various sites, listed in Table 9.1.

This table is by no means exhaustive, but illustrates the various anatomical sites involved, along with the more common causes.

TEST DESCRIPTIONS/TECHNIQUES

UPRIGHT AND SUPINE VITAL CAPACITY

In those with muscle weakness, expiratory volume is determined more by inspiratory muscle strength and lung and chest wall compliance than expiratory flow limitation. Therefore, forced expiratory manoeuvres such as FEV_1 and FVC have less value in this patient group and may be difficult to perform. However, a vital capacity may be measured reliably in most, using a slower manoeuvre whereby the subject is asked to breathe in as deeply as possible and then to breathe out as far as possible through the spirometer at a comfortable pace. Thus VC is generally preferred to FVC for assessment of muscle strength. Paired measurements of vital capacity (VC), made both in the supine position and upright provide greater sensitivity in detection of diaphragmatic weakness than does measurement upright alone.

Results are expressed as a percentage change and given by the equation:

$$\text{Percentage supine VC reduction} = \frac{\text{Upright VC} - \text{Supine VC}}{\text{Upright VC}} \times 100$$

Table 9.1 Causes of respiratory muscle weakness

Anatomical site	Lesion	Notes and examples
Spinal cord lesion	Trauma Transverse myelitis Disc compression Tumour	Diaphragmatic power may be lost following high-cervical cord lesions. Thoracic cord lesions may cause loss of power in intercostal muscles, most apparent in expiration
Motor nerves	Motor neurone disease (MND)[a]/ amyotrophic lateral sclerosis	An invariable complication of MND, which may occur as the presenting complaint or at a terminal stage
	Poliomyelitis[a] and post-polio syndrome	
	Guillain–Barre syndrome	The most common acute cause of respiratory muscle weakness
	Bilateral phrenic nerve lesion[a]	Brachial neuralgia
	Unilateral phrenic nerve lesion	Often asymptomatic, but may cause dyspnoea on exertion. Causes as above plus complications of cardiac surgery or neck surgery, tumour
	Sarcoidosis	May cause a peripheral neuropathy
	Hereditary sensorimotor neuropathy	

(Continued)

Table 9.1 (*Continued*) Causes of respiratory muscle weakness.

Anatomical site	Lesion	Notes and examples
	Critical illness polyneuropathy	May cause difficulty weaning from mechanical ventilation
Neuromuscular junction	Myasthenia gravis	Respiratory involvement is a feature of myasthenic crisis
	Lambert–Eaton syndrome	Respiratory involvement may occur in late stage disease
	Botulism	Typically starts with cranial nerve palsies and descends
	Medication	Neuromuscular blocking agents, aminoglycosides
	Organophosphate poisoning	Found in insecticides and chemical weapons, e.g. Sarin
Muscles	Acid maltase deficiency[a]	Respiratory failure an early finding, presents in young adults
	Mitochondrial myopathy	
	Muscular dystrophy	Duchenne, Becker, fascio-scapulo-humeral, spinal muscular atrophy
	Dystrophia myotonica[a]	
	Polymyositis/ dermatomyositis	Creatine kinase (CK) elevated >1000

[a] Respiratory failure may be a presenting feature of these diseases.

STATIC LUNG VOLUMES

Static lung volumes are not particularly helpful in the assessment of suspected muscle weakness, although certain patterns of abnormality may suggest this diagnosis. The loss of VC is usually offset to some extent by an increase in residual volume (RV), particularly if there is weakness of expiratory muscles. Therefore, the reduction in total lung capacity (TLC) is usually less than that of VC. By contrast to the restrictive defect seen in interstitial lung disease, the RV is usually slightly raised, or unchanged.

MAXIMAL EXPIRATORY PRESSURE

The maximal expiratory pressure (MEP) measures the strength of the abdominal and other expiratory muscles. Simple portable mouth pressure meters are available, although a lab-based system allows for display of the pressure wave on a monitor. To perform the test, a maximal inspiration is taken followed by a maximal expiratory effort against a closed shutter. Effort should continue for at least 1.5 seconds, during which time the highest pressure which can be maintained continuously over 1 second should be recorded. Several efforts should be made to achieve consistent technique and results. An effective mouth seal is essential to prevent pressure loss, and the test may be performed with the patient supporting their cheeks with the flat of their hands, to prevent pressure being dissipated within the buccal cavity. This test is volitional and non-invasive, and the equipment required is affordable, but results tend to be less reproducible than VC measurements. The result is expressed either in cmH_2O or kPa.

MAXIMAL INSPIRATORY PRESSURE

This measures the global strength of the diaphragm and other inspiratory muscles. The patient first expires at a natural pace to RV, and then inspires maximally against the closed shutter. Again, sufficient attempts should be made to achieve repeatable results. The pressure measured during inspiratory tests is expressed as a negative value.

SNIFF NASAL INSPIRATORY PRESSURE

This test provides an assessment of global inspiratory muscle strength. By contrast to maximal inspiratory pressure (MIP), it measures ballistic rather than sustained inspiratory strength. The patient inserts a nasal bung into one nostril, through which a thin catheter is connected to a pressure transducer. The subject performs a sharp maximal sniff from functional residual capacity (FRC), through the opposite nostril. The catheter then measures the pressure within the nasal cavity and upper airway.

This test may be preferred for patients with orofacial weakness, who are unable to maintain a good lip seal around the mouthpiece needed for MIP and MEP. In the presence of obstructive airways disease, transmission of negative pressure across the lungs from the pleura to the transducer may be dampened, so that an under-reading (less negative) is made in subjects with chronic obstructive pulmonary disease (COPD).

SNIFF TRANS-DIAPHRAGMATIC PRESSURE

Inflatable balloon catheters are passed through the nose, one into the oesophagus and one into the stomach. Each contains a pressure transducer. Volitional sniff pressures may then be measured directly across the diaphragm by assessing the pressure difference between the two catheters (Sniff P_{di}). Alternatively, measurements may be made from the oesophageal catheter in isolation, which gives an index of global inspiratory muscle strength.

DIRECT ELECTROMAGNETIC PHRENIC NERVE STIMULATION

This is the gold standard test of diaphragmatic strength (twitch P_{di}). The diaphragm is stimulated directly, providing a non-volitional measure of diaphragmatic muscle strength. This is achieved by phrenic nerve stimulation, using powerful electromagnets placed on each side of the neck. The stimulation is supramaximal to ensure a maximal non-volitional muscular contraction. The procedure is painless, though an uncomfortable sensation. This technique requires specialist equipment and expertise, and therefore is only performed at referral centres.

COUGH PEAK FLOW

The cough peak flow is the velocity of air leaving the respiratory tract during a cough manoeuvre, usually from maximum inspiration. The ability to cough requires coordinated use of inspiratory, bulbar, and expiratory muscles. Adequate cough is essential for clearance of respiratory secretions, particularly during intercurrent infection.

The subject is instructed to breathe in, and then cough into a pneumotachograph or simply a peak flow meter. A mouthpiece may be used as the interface, or alternatively a facemask if it provides a better seal. Several maximal attempts should be made, of which the highest value is recorded. Healthy adults have a cough peak flow of >400 L/min.

ARTERIAL BLOOD GASES

Daytime hypercapnia occurs late in the course of respiratory muscle weakness, and is preceded by nocturnal hypercapnia, which may be suspected on a conventional sleep study by the presence of hypoxia and/or periods of prolonged hypoventilation. A sleep study in which transcutaneous CO_2 is measured is useful in providing confirmation of nocturnal hypoventilation. In patients with incipient hypercapnia, limited to the sleep period, a rise in daytime arterial bicarbonate may provide an early indication of nocturnal hypercapnia before daytime hypercapnia occurs.

PITFALL

In patients with acute neuromuscular failure, arterial blood gases may remain misleadingly normal until respiratory arrest is imminent and so should not be relied upon for reassurance.

RADIOLOGICAL ASSESSMENT OF MUSCLE STRENGTH

The appearance of small lungs on the chest x-ray may provide a clue to the presence of respiratory muscle weakness.

PITFALL

The finding of small lung fields is often overlooked in those with neuromuscular weakness, being mistakenly attributed to poor radiographic technique under those circumstances.

If the diaphragm is paralysed, it moves paradoxically in respiration, being sucked upwards into the thorax by the low pressure created during inspiration. This may be visualised by ultrasound.

However, many patients with diaphragmatic paralysis learn to contract the abdominal muscles during expiration, displacing the diaphragm caudally.

Then, at the start of inspiration, the subject relaxes the abdominal musculature, allowing passive descent of the diaphragm, which may give a misleading radiological picture. This renders radiological assessment of muscle strength rather insensitive and it probably adds little to the assessment made by functional measurements as above.

CLINICAL INTERPRETATION OF TESTS OF MUSCLE STRENGTH

The reference ranges for MIP, MEP, and sniff nasal inspiratory pressure (SNIP) are wide, making comparison to predicted values less useful than with other tests of respiratory function. Moreover, the muscle strength required to maintain adequate ventilation is small, and therefore values which are somewhat low may not be clinically significant. Table 9.2 displays the threshold values of significant abnormality for a variety of respiratory muscle function tests.

MIP, MEP, SNIP, and supine VC all provide slightly different and complementary information about the respiratory musculature and should be interpreted in conjunction with each other.

Where chronic airflow limitation coexists, pulmonary hyperexpansion may be associated with flattening of the diaphragm, under which circumstances it works at a mechanical disadvantage. Therefore, subjects with hyperexpanded lungs may record less negative pressures on any of the tests of inspiratory or diaphragmatic function, despite having normal diaphragmatic contractility.

FORCED VITAL CAPACITY

The VC is often reduced in patients with weakness of the respiratory muscles, which is one cause of a restrictive defect. In the upright posture, the weight of the abdominal viscera aids their descent under the force of the contracting

Table 9.2 Clinically significant values for commonly performed tests of respiratory muscle strength

Respiratory muscle test	Clinically significant muscle weakness
MIP	> -8 kPa (> -3 kPa suggests impending respiratory failure)
MEP	< 8 kPa
Sniff pressure	> -6 kPa
Sniff P_{di}	Male < 0.98 kPa; female < 0.69 kPa

diaphragm. By contrast, when positioned supine the inertia of the abdominal contents opposes the inspiratory movement of the diaphragm. Thus, supine positioning allows testing of diaphragmatic strength under conditions of modest loading.

Therefore, greater sensitivity is gained by making paired readings of VC, in the upright and supine positions. It is generally said that measurement of a normal supine VC, with no significant drop from upright to supine, excludes clinically important weakness of the respiratory muscles as a cause of dyspnoea.

However, a drop in VC upright to supine may be seen in other causes of respiratory disease, and indeed normal subjects. A mean drop of 7.5% (SD ± 5) was seen in a population of normal subjects, with a drop of 11% (±13) in patients with obstructive lung disease and 8% (±8) in patients with restrictive lung disease.[27] Likewise, a drop in supine VC may be seen in subjects with cachexia, malnutrition, and obesity. Therefore, false positives may be seen and the clinician should take into account coexisting lung disease when interpreting the results. Nonetheless, a drop of greater than 12% in normal subjects or greater than 25% in those with significant coexisting lung disease is highly suspicious for diaphragmatic weakness. A lesser drop is non-reassuring and may prompt further investigation.

This test is reproducible in most subjects, non-invasive, easy to perform, and by far the most accessible index of diaphragm dysfunction.

SNIFF NASAL INSPIRATORY PRESSURE

This test may be easier for subjects with orofacial weakness, though underreading may occur in patients with COPD. A sniff nasal pressure more negative than −6 kPa excludes clinically important respiratory muscle weakness. This test is very useful.

MIP AND MEP

MIP and MEP may be difficult to perform, so that erroneously low readings occur in a fair number of patients.

Greater specificity is gained if both the MIP and SNIP are measured, as a normal value of either is reassuring.[28] Normality of MEP when both MIP and SNIP are reduced suggests isolated inspiratory muscle weakness, which is most likely to be diaphragmatic in origin. Isolated expiratory muscle weakness is rare.

Values of MEP above 8 kPa and values of MIP more negative than –8 kPa exclude clinically important respiratory muscle weakness.

THE TWITCH P_{DI}

This provides the gold standard measurement of diaphragmatic strength and is useful in assessment of complex problems, e.g. in polymyositis, which may cause both pulmonary fibrosis and myopathy. It may also be helpful in assessing breathlessness in patients with equivocal or unexplained results from other tests of muscle strength.

SLEEP, VENTILATORY FAILURE, AND VC

Arterial P_{CO_2} may rise by approximately 0.5 kPa during sleep in normal subjects, due to a number of factors. These include the additional load placed upon the diaphragm when supine and hypotonia of the intercostal muscles during rapid eye movement (REM) sleep. This rise in arterial CO_2 is accompanied by a commensurate drop in arterial P_{O_2}. In those whose respiratory musculature is weakened by disease, much greater accumulation of CO_2 may occur overnight, with periods of deleterious hypoxia.

The progressive course of chronic neuromuscular disease is associated with a typical progressive pattern of sleep disordered breathing, which parallels the decline in VC.[29] The natural history of this course of events leads from sleep disordered breathing through daytime hypercapnia to cor pulmonale and ultimately mortality, if untreated (Table 9.3).

Sleep-disordered breathing is the first manifestation of incipient ventilatory failure and may be identified by the following findings, evident during a sleep study:

Table 9.3 Correlation between IVC and development of ventilatory failure

Supine IVC	Sleep study findings
<60%	Hypopnoeas, especially during REM sleep
<40%	Longer periods of hypoventilation, especially during, but not limited to, REM sleep
<25%	Daytime hypercapnia

Abbreviations: IVC, inspiratory vital capacity; REM, rapid eye movement.

Hypopnoeas are defined as reductions in the amplitude of breathing of >30% (measured by airflow through the mouth or nose), lasting for >10 seconds and associated with a drop in peripheral saturation of >3% (Figure 9.1).[30] These brief interruptions of breathing are most commonly seen in patients with sleep apnoea, in which case they are obstructive in origin, caused by transient occlusion of the upper airway during sleep. However, they may also be seen in patients with neuromuscular weakness, in which case they are central rather than obstructive in origin, relating to abnormality of ventilatory control in those with incipient ventilatory failure.

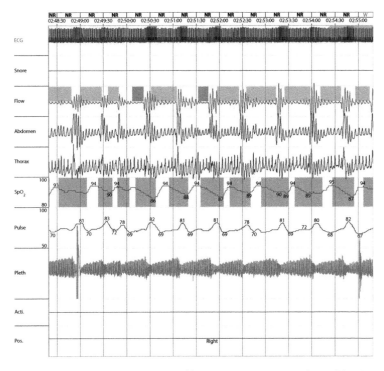

Figure 9.1 Hypopnoea. A cluster of hypopnoeas is seen, indicated by the lighter shade bars on the airflow signal (top line). During these events the airflow diminishes, but does not stop. By contrast, apnoeas are marked with a darker bar. Each vertical deflection of the signal trace on the flow channel represents a single breath. Oxygenation dips during each hypopnoea (S_pO_2, sixth line). Thoracoabdominal movements continue (Abdomen and Thorax, fourth and fifth lines). During these events, airflow stops. Each vertical bar on the y-axis represents 30 seconds of time.

Hypoventilation may be defined as an increase in transcutaneous CO_2 to a value of 7.3 kPa (55 mmHg), sustained for >10 minutes.[30] Although rigorous classification of hypoventilation requires measurement of transcutaneous CO_2, hypoventilation may also be inferred by identification of prolonged periods of hypopnoea, during which there is a sustained drop in S_pO_2 (Figure 9.2).

Hypopnoeas may occur in subjects with early neuromuscular disease, but are initially restricted to periods of REM sleep, due to the hypotonia of skeletal

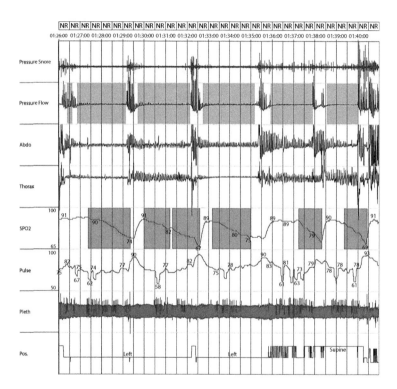

Figure 9.2 Hypoventilation. Very prolonged periods of hypopnoea are indicated by the shaded bars in the nasal airflow channel. This sample is compressed on the time axis, to show the longer events, though each vertical bar on the *y*-axis still represents 30 seconds of time. Each vertical deflection on the pressure flow channel represents a single breath. It is seen that the amplitude of breathing is markedly reduced during these prolonged hypopnoeas. The duration of each of these events is >2.5 minutes. They are associated with deep desaturation to below 70% (indicated shaded bars, S_pO_2 channel). Thoracoabdominal movement continues, but is diminished. The events occur in both the left lateral and supine positions (position channel, bottom).

musculature which accompanies REM sleep (Figure 9.3). In later-stage disease, these hypopnoeic events lengthen into long periods of hypoventilation during REM sleep. Subsequently, these periods of hypoventilation appear throughout both REM and non-REM sleep. Paradoxically, the measured apnoea/hypopnoea index (total events per hour) may reduce with worsening severity, as the greater length of the events causes a reciprocal reduction in their frequency. Ultimately, daytime hypercapnia supervenes.

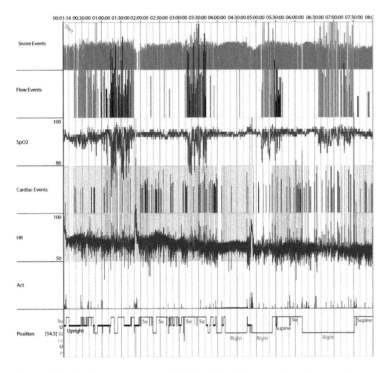

Figure 9.3 Rapid eye movement (REM)-related desaturation. The graphs are summary data from a whole night's sleep. Each vertical bar on the y-axis represents 10 minutes of time. Although this study is not performed with electroencephalogram (EEG) monitoring to allow formal sleep staging, the timing of REM sleep may be inferred from the periodic desaturations which are evident on the S_pO_2 channel. Typically, REM sleep first occurs 90 minutes after sleep-onset and subsequently at 90-minute intervals throughout the remainder of the sleep period. The duration of an episode of REM sleep is typically around 20 minutes. The periods during which profound desaturation are visible in the above trace match that distribution.

Thus, during the course of progressive myopathy, nocturnal hypoventilation precedes the onset of daytime ventilatory failure. Morning headaches provide a symptomatic warning of the night-time's events, caused by cerebral vasodilation, secondary to nocturnal hypercapnia. These headaches characteristically resolve within the first few minutes of the day as hypercapnia dissipates after awakening. Daytime somnolence is caused by the deleterious effect of the repeated respiratory events, which cause continual arousal from deep sleep. If these symptoms are not identified, then the course of ventilatory failure progresses to ascending oedema and the syndrome of cor pulmonale. Finally, patients may present emergently with high elevation of P_{CO_2} (e.g. >10 kPa), severe respiratory acidosis, and coma.

Cor pulmonale refers to the accumulation of dependent oedema in the context of ventilatory failure. Although classically attributed to right ventricular failure, the progression of oedema correlates more closely with daytime CO_2 accumulation than right ventricular function and is more likely attributable to neurohumoral mechanisms than right ventricular mechanics. Historically, cor pulmonale was a terminal development for those with muscle disease, though the advent of non-invasive domiciliary ventilatory support has now increased longevity, particularly for patients with slowly progressive congenital dystrophies.

Reduction of VC is also predictive of the tendency to chest infections, shown in children and adolescents with various myopathies.[31]

CLINICAL PEARLS

GUILLAIN–BARRÉ SYNDROME

Guillain–Barré syndrome is the commonest cause of acute neuromuscular disease and may progress to life-threatening respiratory failure in around 20% of cases, who then require mechanical ventilatory support. Vital capacity is the best bedside means of monitoring the progression of respiratory muscle impairment in this condition and should be measured regularly in all patients, to warn of impending respiratory failure. Measurement of peak flow is not particularly helpful in this scenario. A vital capacity of at least 15 mL/kg is required to maintain spontaneous ventilation, and a drop to less than this is an indication for intubation and mechanical ventilation. Ventilation should be considered earlier if the patient is tiring or if there is pharyngeal in-coordination such that the airway is poorly maintained.

DAYTIME HYPERCAPNIA

The slightest elevation of arterial P_{CO_2} above 6.5 kPa is predictive of acute decompensated ventilatory failure, in subjects with neuromuscular disease. This is by contrast to patients with COPD, who may exist in a relatively stable state with chronic elevation of arterial CO_2. This finding in a patient with neuromuscular disease should prompt urgent referral, whether symptomatic or not.

SNIFF NASAL INSPIRATORY PRESSURE

Sniff inspiratory pressure is more sensitive than either MIP or VC in detection of early respiratory muscle weakness in patients with motor neurone disease.[32] Moreover, this index provides greater linearity in tracking decline of respiratory muscle strength in this group of patients. A SNIP less negative than −4 kPa is predictive of significant nocturnal hypoxia.[33] Both a SNIP value less negative than −4 kPa and an FVC <50% normal were predictive of mortality at 6 months in patients with motor neurone disease, with the SNIP being the more predictive of the two.[33]

By contrast, VC best predicts respiratory failure, tendency to infection and survival in those with congenital myopathies and dystrophies. However, SNIP may be easier to perform by some subjects, particularly children. (Summarised[34]).

MAXIMAL INSPIRATORY PRESSURE

MIP also correlates closely with VC and accordingly is also predictive of nocturnal and daytime hypercapnia. An MIP of less than one-third normal predicts the presence of daytime hypercapnia in patients with motor neurone disease, but is less predictive than SNIP.[32]

COUGH PEAK FLOW

Inadequate cough may be problematic for any patient with ventilatory muscle weakness, particularly in those with significant involvement of expiratory muscles, e.g. spinal muscular atrophy. Cough peak flow is an important determinant of susceptibility to chest infections, which account for both morbidity and mortality in patients with severe muscle weakness.

A cough peak flow of less than 270 L/min in an adolescent or adult, measured when well, indicates vulnerability to respiratory failure during chest infections, due to inability to clear sputum. A cough peak flow <160 L/min indicates that cough is profoundly weak. Extubation or decannulation of ventilated patients whose cough peak flow is <160 L/min is prone to failure, but may be achieved by very careful use of non-invasive ventilation (NIV) and assisted cough techniques, including insufflator/exsufflator devices.

An MEP of <6 kPa also predicts a weak cough in patients with muscular dystrophy.[35]

SPINAL CORD INJURY

Paradoxically, patients with low cervical cord injuries (C4–C7) experience greater loss of VC in the sitting position than when supine.[36]

KEY POINTS/SUMMARY

- Respiratory muscle weakness is often unsuspected and may be missed until a patient decompensates and presents emergently, in extreme ventilatory failure.
- Hypercapnia in those with muscle weakness is often mistakenly attributed to COPD.
- A supine reduction in vital capacity may be useful in identifying inspiratory muscle weakness and diaphragmatic paralysis.

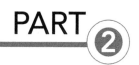

PART 2

BLOOD GAS INTERPRETATION

10

Assessment of ventilation

INTRODUCTION

Ventilation refers to the rate at which air is breathed in and out of the lungs. Alveolar ventilation is a parameter of fundamental importance, as it is the primary determinant of arterial CO_2 concentration. Arterial P_{CO_2} is a key factor in determining arterial P_{O_2}, making it helpful to consider CO_2 before looking at oxygenation.

MEASURED INDICES/KEY DEFINITIONS

Table 10.1 shows various parameters which are relevant to ventilation.

Although each breath contains around 500 mL, approximately 150 mL do not reach the alveoli but remain within the dead space, which is comprised of the trachea and major airways.

The minute volume of ventilation ($\dot{V}_E$) is the volume of air breathed per minute. This is more conveniently measured, and therefore normally expressed as the expired volume. In normal individuals, this is approximately 7 L/min at rest.

The minute volume of alveolar ventilation ($\dot{V}_A$) is the volume of air breathed per minute which actually reaches the gas-exchanging area of the lungs, i.e. the minute volume of ventilation less the volume which goes in and out of the dead space each minute.

PHYSIOLOGY OF VENTILATION IN RELATION TO CO_2

From the definitions given above, alveolar ventilation may be expressed as

$$\dot{V}_A = \text{Respiratory rate} \times (V_T - V_D)$$

Table 10.1 Various parameters relevant to ventilation

Abbreviation	Parameter	Definition/comment
V_T	Tidal volume	Volume of air in each breath
V_D	Dead space	Volume of air in each breath which does not reach alveoli
V_A	Alveolar volume	Volume of air in each breath which does reach the alveoli
$\dot{V}_E$	Minute volume of ventilation	Volume of air breathed each minute (exhaled)
$\dot{V}_A$	Minute volume of alveolar ventilation	Volume of air breathed per minute, which reaches the gas-exchanging area of the lungs.
$\dot{V}_{CO_2}$	Rate of production of CO_2	
P_aCO_2	Partial pressure of CO_2 in arterial blood	
P_vCO_2	Partial pressure of CO_2 in peripheral venous blood	

Therefore at rest, with a respiratory rate of 15:

$$\dot{V}_A = 15 \times (500 - 150)$$
$$5.25 \text{ L/min}$$

CO_2 is produced in the tissues, from where it is carried by the circulation to the alveoli. This alveolar CO_2 is continuously diluted into the volume of air passing through the alveoli, by the process of ventilation. Therefore, intuitively the alveolar CO_2 concentration is the ratio of total body CO_2 production to the minute volume of alveolar ventilation:

$$\text{Alveolar } CO_2 \text{ concentration} = \frac{\dot{V}_{CO_2}}{\dot{V}_A}$$

CO_2 is highly soluble in physical solution and its passage from the pulmonary capillaries to alveoli is not limited by the efficiency of ventilation–perfusion matching. Therefore, arterial P_{CO_2} is approximately equal to alveolar P_{CO_2}:

$$\text{Arterial } P_{CO_2} \approx \frac{\dot{V}_{CO_2}}{\dot{V}_A}$$

Thus, we have an equation which predicts the approximate value of arterial P_{CO_2}. From this relationship, we can understand that arterial P_{CO_2} is inversely proportional to the minute volume of ventilation.

KEY POINTS

- Ventilatory failure occurs when the minute volume of alveolar ventilation is insufficient to keep pace with the rate of CO_2 production, so that P_{CO_2} rises above 6.5 kPa.
- If we double our respiratory rate, we will halve the arterial P_{CO_2} (all other things remaining equal).
- Type 2 respiratory failure is synonymous with ventilatory failure.

Although the relationship above shows that hypercapnia may be caused by either under-ventilation or overproduction of CO_2, in practice a raised P_{CO_2} is invariably caused by under-ventilation, so that arterial P_{CO_2} is an index of ventilatory sufficiency. Only occasionally does increased production of CO_2 contribute to hypercapnia. Table 10.2 lists a range of causes of ventilatory failure.

Table 10.2 Causes of hypercapnia

	Condition	Comment
Airways disease	COPD	Classically the 'blue bloater' subtype is hypercapnic. Emphysematous destruction of alveoli results in dead space, but COPD patients also hypoventilate with a tolerance of hypercapnia which is poorly understood
	Asthma	Rising P_{CO_2} is a sign of impending respiratory arrest
	Upper airway obstruction	Reduction of luminal diameter may increase airway resistance to the point where minute ventilation cannot be maintained against the work of breathing. A raised P_{CO_2} in this context is a late sign and respiratory arrest may soon follow

(Continued)

Table 10.2 (*Continued*) Causes of hypercapnia

	Condition	Comment
Chest wall disorder	Obesity hypoventilation syndrome	Adiposity creates additional loading of the thoracic wall, with resultant low minute volume. This is a common cause of a chronic hypercapnia
	Neuromuscular disease	Motor neurone disease, bilateral diaphragmatic paralysis, muscular dystrophy, myopathy
	Reduced chest wall compliance	Post-thoracoplasty, kyphoscoliosis, hide-bound chest of scleroderma
	Loss of structural integrity	Flail chest
Central depression of respiratory drive		Drugs, e.g. opioids, benzodiazepines, anaesthetic agents
		Brainstem lesion
Exhaustion		Any cause of acute respiratory distress especially if associated with increased work of breathing, e.g. asthma, acute pulmonary oedema

Because of the very large volume of CO_2 (around 120 L) held buffered in the body, it takes 20–30 minutes for a new steady state to be reached after a change in ventilation. In a situation of total respiratory arrest, P_{CO_2} rises by only about 0.4–0.8 kPa/min. By contrast, total body oxygen content is much lower (around 1.5 L whilst breathing air), and P_{O_2} equilibrates within a minute or two of any change in the rate of ventilation.

NORMAL VALUES

- P_aCO_2 – At rest, alveolar ventilation is adjusted to maintain P_aCO_2 close to 5.2 kPa in healthy subjects. It is not influenced by age. A P_aCO_2 >6.5 kPa indicates significant abnormality and defines type 2 respiratory failure.
- $\dot{V}_E$ – At rest, the normal minute volume of ventilation is around 7 L/min.

MEASUREMENT OF VENOUS BLOOD GASES

There is increasing interest in the use of venous blood gases for monitoring of P_{CO_2} and pH in patients with acute respiratory failure, as these values correlate somewhat to the respective arterial values.

This subject has been examined by meta-analysis,[37] which has been helpful in collating the disparate results.

The peripheral venous pH is approximately 0.03 lower than that of arterial blood, with 95% confidence intervals lying approximately 0.1 either side. For example, a venous pH of 7.3 probably indicates an arterial pH of 7.33, but could indicate an arterial pH of anywhere between 7.23 and 7.43.

Likewise, the peripheral venous P_{CO_2} is approximately 0.75 ± 3 kPa higher than that of arterial blood. For example, a venous P_{CO_2} of 7 kPa probably indicates an arterial P_{CO_2} of 6.25 kPa, but the arterial value may lie anywhere between 3.25 and 9.25 kPa. Surprisingly, the peripheral venous P_{CO_2} may be higher or lower than that measured in arterial P_{CO_2}.

Venous bicarbonate is 1.3 ± 3 kPa mmol/L higher than arterial (The normal range of arterial bicarbonate varies between manufacturers of blood gas analysis equipment, but is typically 22–26 mmol/L.)

In summary:

- Venous pH is a useful surrogate for arterial pH, to the extent that a normal venous pH makes significant respiratory acidosis unlikely.
- Venous P_{CO_2} is unreliable as a surrogate for arterial P_{CO_2}.
- If the venous pH and bicarbonate are both normal, then significant acidosis or hypercapnia are unlikely.

Therefore, venous blood gases may be a useful screening measure which avoids arterial puncture, but if either the venous pH or bicarbonate suggest abnormality, arterial blood gases should be measured.

CAUSES OF HYPERCAPNIA

Hypoventilation of gas-exchanging alveoli is the commonest mechanism of hypercapnia. Dead space may be raised and/or minute ventilation reduced (see Table 10.2).

PITFALL

Although chronic obstructive pulmonary disease (COPD) is by far the commonest cause of hypercapnia, familiarity with this condition frequently leads doctors to miss other causes of hypercapnia.

CHRONIC OBSTRUCTIVE PULMONARY DISEASE

A subgroup of patients with COPD are prone to chronic hypercapnia. This subtype has been termed 'blue bloaters' in distinction to their counterparts, 'pink puffers' who maintain normal P_{CO_2}. The determinants of this dichotomy are unclear, though it does not appear to reflect disease severity. Many pink puffers will reach end-stage disease without becoming blue bloaters. Nonetheless, chronic CO_2 retention in patients with COPD confers a worse prognosis overall.

Supplemental oxygen therapy may precipitate hypercapnia in those prone to CO_2 retention. It is generally believed that hypercapnic patients rely upon hypoxia to stimulate their respiratory drive. Thus, it is postulated that when surplus oxygen is administered, hypoventilation results. However, this belief is not strongly supported by the evidence available, which has shown no depression of minute ventilation in response to supplemental oxygen amongst patients with COPD.[38] Rather, it appears that supplemental oxygen abolishes hypoxic vasoconstriction in poorly ventilated areas of the lung and so increases dead space.

KEY POINTS

- It should be emphasised that most patients who present acutely to hospital with hypoxia, caused by conditions such as asthma, pneumonia, pulmonary oedema, or pulmonary embolism are in no danger of CO_2 retention. High-concentration oxygen is immediately life-saving and should never be withheld needlessly.
- Patients who are at risk of CO_2 retention are usually readily identifiable by the history and examination findings of severe COPD; only in this group should oxygen concentration be carefully controlled.
- Importantly, hypoxia kills patients quickly, whereas hypercapnia kills patients slowly. Therefore, if doubt exists about the appropriateness of administering high-concentration oxygen therapy, it is preferable to do so in order to treat hypoxia, until further information becomes available from blood gas measurement or otherwise.

During exacerbations of COPD, caution should be applied when administering supplemental oxygen to patients who are prone to CO_2 retention, as the development of hypercapnia confers significant excess mortality under these circumstances.[39] Oxygen should initially be administered in a concentration of 24%–28%, targeted to an S_pO_2 of 88%–92%. Blood gases should be measured after 30–60 minutes. If the pH is satisfactory, the F_IO_2 may be increased as needed until the P_{O_2} is greater than 7.6 kPa, rechecking blood gases 30–60 minutes after each increment.

If a patient remains acidotic despite medical management, acute treatment with non-invasive ventilation may be life-saving.

OBESITY HYPOVENTILATION SYNDROME

This is a severe form of sleep disordered breathing, usually occurring in the markedly obese, in whom increased chest wall loading results in nocturnal hypoventilation and ultimately daytime hypercapnia. Such patients follow a similar trajectory to those with neuromuscular disease, but without such close correlation to forced vital capacity (FVC) (see 'Sleep, ventilatory failure, and FVC' in Chapter 9).

Patients with obesity-hypoventilation syndrome (OHS) almost invariably have coexisting obstructive sleep apnoea, though a small proportion may have nocturnal hypoventilation in isolation.

In healthy individuals, P_{CO_2} rises during sleep by around 0.5 kPa, but may rise to 12–13 kPa in those with OHS. The symptom of morning headache, caused by CO_2 retention overnight is characteristic. The diagnosis may be confirmed by a polysomnographic sleep study, ideally with transcutaneous monitoring of P_{CO_2}.

The treatment of OHS is with non-invasive ventilation or continuous positive airway pressure (CPAP), according to severity. Typical treatment equipment is illustrated in Figure 7.1.

EXHAUSTION

Arterial P_{CO_2} may rise in any patient with respiratory failure who becomes exhausted and therefore unable to maintain adequate ventilatory effort. This may occur in acute asthma or pulmonary oedema, in both of which the work of breathing may be increased to an unsustainable level.

Patients in this situation are gravely ill. Lack of respiratory drive is not the problem, and despite the high P_{CO_2}, high concentration and flow oxygen should be given whilst definitive management is commenced. Brief apnoeas or sudden reductions in respiratory rate are a sign of *imminent respiratory arrest*.

INCREASED CO_2 PRODUCTION

High production of CO_2 may contribute to a raised P_{CO_2}. This is uncommon, but a feature of malignant hyperthermia, a severe reaction which may occur following administration of certain anaesthetic drugs.

CAUSES OF LOW P_{CO_2}

In clinical practice, hypocapnia is less of a problem than raised P_{CO_2}. Various causes are listed below.

HYPOXAEMIA

A low arterial P_{O_2}, especially when less than 7 kPa, causes an increase in ventilatory drive, with a consequent reduction in P_{CO_2} (see 'Relationship between alveolar P_{O_2} and arterial P_{CO_2}' in Chapter 12).

METABOLIC ACIDOSIS

A metabolic acidosis causes an increase in ventilatory drive, such that the reduction in arterial P_{CO_2} compensates the acidosis.

CENTRAL NERVOUS SYSTEM DISORDERS

Subarachnoid haemorrhage, infarction, and infection may cause hyperventilation by cerebral irritation or direct effect upon the respiratory centre in the midbrain.

DRUGS

Salicylates and progestogens stimulate respiratory drive, tending to cause a low P_{CO_2}.

ANXIETY

Anxiety or psychological trauma may provoke severe hyperventilation. It is important to exclude other causes before making this diagnosis. Under conditions of hyperventilation, a rise in P_{O_2} should be seen which is commensurate with the depression of P_{CO_2} (see 'Relationship between alveolar P_{O_2} and arterial P_{CO_2}' in Chapter 12).

CLINICAL PEARLS

- Respiratory regulation of arterial P_{CO_2} is tightly controlled. Even the slightest elevation above 6.5 kPa indicates significant abnormality.
- Many patients with COPD have a persistently raised arterial P_{CO_2} of up to 9 kPa or more which is surprisingly well tolerated. If this is long-standing, it may be compensated, that is the pH is normal. P_{CO_2} must always be read in conjunction with pH.
- In patients with neuromuscular disease, an arterial P_{CO_2} which is >6.5 kPa is a grave sign that decompensated ventilatory failure may be imminent.
- A patient becomes comatose when P_{CO_2} reaches 12–16 kPa, though neurological impairment correlates better with cerebrospinal fluid pH than arterial P_{CO_2}.
- In patients with COPD, both FEV_1 and chronic hypercapnia are independent predictors of mortality.
- Correlation between FEV_1 and the development of hypercapnia is poor in patients with COPD, though hypercapnia is uncommon in those with an FEV_1 >1 L or >50% predicted.
- The characteristic clinical signs of hypercapnia, i.e. venous dilatation, bounding pulse, flap (asterixis), papilloedema, and confusion, are unreliable and frequently absent.
- Many new presentations of neuromuscular disease are initially misdiagnosed as COPD on first assessment in the emergency department, on the basis of hypercapnia.
- COPD is an unlikely cause of ventilatory failure in anyone under 50 years of age or anyone who has a smoking history of less than 40 pack-years. A diagnosis of COPD under these circumstances is to be questioned.

KEY POINTS/SUMMARY

- Adequacy of ventilation is assessed by the measurement of arterial P_{CO_2} during arterial blood gas analysis.
- Ventilatory failure is due to inadequate ventilation of gas-exchanging alveoli.
- The minute volume of ventilation is inversely proportional to the arterial P_{CO_2}.
- P_aCO_2 >6.5 kPa defines type 2 respiratory failure, which is synonymous with ventilatory failure.

11

Assessment of haemoglobin saturation

INTRODUCTION

Haemoglobin saturation can be measured directly by arterial blood gas analysis, but is more conveniently measured by the use of a pulse oximeter. Arterial oxygenation correlates with the arterial oxygen tension (P_aO_2), in a relationship described by the familiar S-shaped oxygen dissociation curve (Figure 11.1). Because of its ease of measurement, reduced peripheral saturation is often the first indication of respiratory failure.

MEASURED INDICES

Table 11.1 shows the various parameters relevant to blood oxygenation.

$\dot{D}O_2$ is the rate at which oxygen is delivered to the tissues, given by the product of arterial blood oxygen concentration and cardiac output. (See 'What determines the amount of oxygen carried in blood?' below.)

$\dot{V}O_2$ is the rate at which oxygen is consumed by tissue metabolism, which in a normal resting subject approximates one quarter of that delivered, leaving a substantial reserve within the blood which may be drawn upon under conditions of stress.

S_vO_2 is the mixed venous saturation, measured from blood taken from the right ventricular outflow tract or pulmonary artery. As different tissues vary widely in their oxygen utilisation, venous blood returning from different regions of the body differs widely in its oxygen saturation. However, the venous return from the whole body is mixed during its passage through the right heart, so that blood oxygenation within the right ventricular outflow tract or pulmonary artery provides an overall index of oxygen utilisation. Although this blood is not readily accessible for measurement, the parameter is important conceptually.

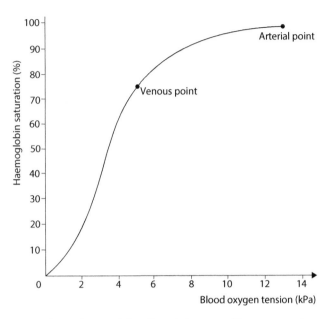

Figure 11.1 The oxyhaemoglobin dissociation curve. The venous point represents the oxygenation of mixed venous blood.

Table 11.1 Parameters relevant to blood oxygenation

Symbol	Description
S_aO_2	Arterial haemoglobin oxygen saturation (%, measured *in vitro*)
S_pO_2	Arterial haemoglobin oxygen saturation (%, measured by pulse oximetry)
C_aO_2	Arterial oxygen concentration (mL/L)
$\dot{D}O_2$	Oxygen delivery to the tissues per minute (mL/min)
$\dot{V}O_2$	Rate of oxygen consumption by tissue metabolism (mL/min)
$S_{\bar{v}}O_2$	Mixed venous oxygen saturation (%, measured on blood from the right ventricular outflow tract or pulmonary artery)

MEASUREMENT OF OXYGEN SATURATION

S_aO_2 may be measured directly during arterial blood gas analysis. Although this remains the gold standard means of measurement of haemoglobin saturation, arterial puncture is invasive and carries the potential complications of bleeding, trauma, and infection.

PULSE OXIMETRY

Reduced haemoglobin is bluish in colour, giving the hypoxic patient a cyanotic appearance when severe. Well-oxygenated blood is cherry red. Pulse oximetry quantifies arterial blood colour by its light absorption, measured during arterial pulsation. From this, the proportion of haemoglobin combined with oxygen (the oxygen saturation) is derived. The measurement is made non-invasively using a probe attached to the finger, toe, ear lobe or nasal septum. In addition to pulse rate and continuous oxygen saturation, better oximeters display a peripheral pulse waveform.

WAVEFORM

The waveform is important in providing a means of ensuring good transduction of the arterial pulse. A normal waveform has a dicrotic notch on the downslope of the wave, as seen in an arterial pressure waveform (Figure 11.2). Poor transduction may cause loss of the dicrotic notch, loss of signal amplitude, flattening of the waveform, and ultimately erratic loss of trace. Poor transduction of the arterial signal may result from several causes, listed in Table 11.2. Notably, the measurement provided by pulse oximetry is not affected by skin pigmentation.

A low saturation reading should prompt a check of the pulse waveform. If the waveform is poor, then an artefactually low reading may be suspected. Pulse waveform display is a requisite feature of an oximeter used for monitoring of acutely unwell patients.

Pitfall

If low saturation is measured in the presence of a good waveform, real hypoxaemia must be assumed until proven otherwise, and poor transduction should not be implicated.

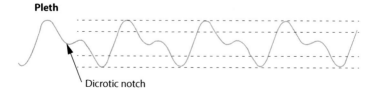

Figure 11.2 The waveform of pulse oximetry.

Table 11.2 Causes of poor pulse oximetry signal likely to cause erroneous measurement of saturation

Cause	Note/comment
Malposition or poor attachment of the probe to the skin	–
Motion artefact	E.g. shivering, agitation.
Poor peripheral circulation	E.g. cold hands, hypothermia, Raynaud's, scleroderma, peripheral vascular disease. Earlobe is better in subjects with poor peripheral circulation.
Low cardiac output	The accuracy of pulse oximetry reduces when the blood pressure drops below 80 mmHg.
Inflation of sphygmomanometer cuff on the same arm as the saturation probe	Use opposite sides for each.

ACCURACY

Pulse oximetry measurement apparatus is calibrated by comparison to measurement of S_aO_2 made on samples of arterial blood, taken from healthy volunteers. In order to calibrate the measurements over a range of values, normal volunteers are given reducing levels of F_IO_2, to achieve resting saturation values of 80%–100%. Calibration below this range is achieved by extrapolation of the above. Manufacturers claim good accuracy from these data, to within 2% over the range 80%–100% and 3% below that.

Nonetheless, studies which have made a comparison between S_pO_2 and S_aO_2 measured in acutely unwell patients have shown significant discrepancies, with S_pO_2 tending to overestimate the true S_aO_2. A study of intensive therapy unit (ITU) patients showed that it was necessary to maintain S_pO_2 at 94% in order to ensure an S_aO_2 of 90%.[40] A more recent study of patients admitted to hospital with acute exacerbations of chronic obstructive pulmonary disease (COPD) found a wide scatter of S_pO_2 in relation to S_aO_2, with 95% confidence intervals of S_aO_2 lying ±10% of S_pO_2.[41]

KEY POINT

Whilst S_pO_2 is invaluable for monitoring patients in acute respiratory failure, this information should be supplemented by occasional arterial blood gas analysis, for measurement of both S_aO_2 and blood gases.

SPECIFIC SOURCES OF ERROR

Misleading results may occur in the presence of congenital or acquired haemoglobin abnormalities.

Carboxyhaemoglobinaemia

Pulse oximetry registers carboxyhaemoglobin as oxyhaemoglobin, so that a misleadingly high measurement of S_pO_2 is made in those exposed to carbon monoxide (see 'Carbon monoxide poisoning').

Methaemoglobinaemia

Methaemoglobinaemia may occur as a hereditary abnormality but is more commonly a result of drug toxicity, particularly caused by administration of local anaesthetic drugs or Dapsone. The presence of methaemoglobin in the circulation imparts an intense blue/grey colour to the skin. Pulse oximetry indicates a low saturation in those with methaemoglobinaemia, despite adequate arterial Po_2. The diagnosis is confirmed by measurement in an arterial blood gas analyser which is equipped to measure methaemoglobin.

Haemoglobinopathy

Several haemoglobin variants may exist at low saturation despite adequate arterial Po_2. These are rare.

Nail varnish

Dark nail varnish or false nails may cause an under-reading of S_pO_2 despite adequate waveform, by their effect upon light absorption. This error may be mitigated by placing the probe on the finger crossways.

PROS AND CONS OF PULSE OXIMETRY

Pulse oximetry offers various advantages over arterial blood gas analysis:

1. Real-time data at the bedside
2. Continuous monitoring, for high-dependency patients and those undergoing anaesthesia
3. Domiciliary monitoring either for spot-checks or continuous sleep study monitoring
4. Non-invasive measurement

However, the following limitations apply:

1. Inability to detect over-oxygenation – a saturation of 98% would be consistent with a Po_2 of 10 or 30 kPa.
2. Lack of information about Pco_2 and therefore ventilatory status. Measurement of arterial blood gases allows calculation of the alveolar–arterial difference (see 'Alveolar–arterial partial pressure Po_2 difference' in Chapter 12).
3. Deviation of S_po_2 from S_ao_2. This is often within acceptable margins, as long as the value of S_po_2 >80%.

PHYSIOLOGY – OXYGEN DISSOCIATION CURVE

The vast majority of circulating O_2 is chemically bound to haemoglobin, unlike CO_2 which exists in blood as a physical solution. The haemoglobin-bound O_2 is in equilibrium with a much smaller pool of oxygen in physical solution. Nonetheless, it is the tension of that in physical solution which is measured by blood gas analysis (P_ao_2).

The relationship between the saturation of haemoglobin and the tension of oxygen in physical solution is non-linear and described by the familiar sigmoidal or S-shaped oxyhaemoglobin dissociation curve (Figure 11.1). Several important characteristics of oxygen transport may be discerned from the properties of the oxyhaemoglobin dissociation curve.

Because the curve has a prolonged plateau at high saturations, haemoglobin saturation is not appreciably reduced by a drop in oxygen tension until P_ao_2 falls below 10 kPa, so that blood oxygen content remains high under conditions of mild-moderate hypoxia. Once on the steeper part of the curve, any further drop in P_ao_2 causes a significant reduction in arterial saturation.

The curve shifts to the right under conditions of acidosis, raised $P_a\text{co}_2$, increased temperature and raised intracellular levels of the intermediary metabolite 2,3-diphosphoglycerate (2,3-DPG). A right shift of the curve promotes the unloading of O_2, making it more available to working tissues.

When haemoglobin is in the tissue capillary circulation, it is exposed to a greater concentration of the acidic gas CO_2. Under these circumstances, there is a further reduction of haemoglobin affinity for oxygen (i.e. it carries less O_2 at the same $P\text{o}_2$). This facilitates unloading of O_2 to the tissues. In the pulmonary circulation, where CO_2 concentration is lower, the curve shifts back to the left, promoting oxygen binding and uptake. This effect of pH on the affinity of oxygen is known as the Bohr effect.

WHAT DETERMINES THE AMOUNT OF OXYGEN CARRIED IN BLOOD?

The total amount of oxygen carried per volume of blood, or oxygen content, is the product of haemoglobin concentration (approximately 15 g/dL), haemoglobin saturation (97% or 0.97) and the oxygen combining capacity of haemoglobin (1.31 mL/g), plus a small contribution of about 0.3 mL/dL from oxygen dissolved in physical solution. Therefore, the normal approximate oxygen carrying capacity is given by

$$\text{Arterial oxygen content} = (15 \times 0.97 \times 1.31) + 0.3 = 19.3 \text{ mL/dL}$$

Oxygen delivery to tissues is the product of oxygen content and cardiac output.

KEY POINT

Haemoglobin saturation in the arterial circulation is determined by arterial $P\text{o}_2$, according to the relationship described by the oxyhaemoglobin dissociation curve. Arterial $P\text{o}_2$ in turn is determined by alveolar $P\text{o}_2$ and the efficiency of gas transfer from the alveoli to the pulmonary capillaries. However, it is the resultant haemoglobin saturation, rather than arterial $P\text{o}_2$, which determines blood oxygen content, and therefore oxygen delivery to the tissues. The adequacy of oxygen delivery to the tissues then in turn determines the intracellular $P\text{o}_2$ on which cellular respiration depends.

NORMAL VALUES

C_aO_2 (arterial oxygen concentration) – Approximately 19 mL/dL, or 190 mL/L.

S_aO_2/S_pO_2 – 96%–99%. Healthy lungs should be efficient enough to fully saturate all normal haemoglobin passing through the pulmonary circulation. Admixture with shunted venous blood from the bronchial circulation and Thebesian veins reduces normal saturation to approximately 97%.

$\dot{D}o_2$–Approximately 1000 mL/min are delivered to tissues at rest.

$\dot{V}o_2$–Approximately 250 mL/min at rest, giving an extraction of approximately 25%. The remaining oxygen provides an important reserve which may be utilised under conditions of increased demand, such as exercise, stress, or illness. Under these circumstances, extraction may rise to around 75%.

$S_{\bar{v}}o_2$ – Approximately 70%–75% at rest. This can drop markedly during periods of increased demand.

CARBON MONOXIDE POISONING

Carbon monoxide intoxication is a common poisoning which should be diagnosed quickly, but is frequently unsuspected. Symptoms are non-specific, requiring a high level of suspicion for recognition, including nausea, vertigo, ataxia, breathlessness, and tachycardia, progressing to confusion, seizures, and coma. A 'cherry red' appearance to the lips is classically described, but uncommonly seen.

Carbon monoxide competes with oxygen for haemoglobin binding sites in the pulmonary circulation, resulting in low arterial oxygen saturation, despite well-maintained arterial Po_2. This occurs because carbon monoxide has an affinity for haemoglobin approximately 240 times greater than that of oxygen, and preferentially displaces oxygen from haemoglobin binding sites.

However, pulse oximetry cannot distinguish between oxyhaemoglobin and carboxyhaemoglobin, giving an erroneously high reading of haemoglobin oxygenation under these circumstances. A direct measurement of S_aO_2 by arterial blood gas analysis is required to make the distinction between oxyhaemoglobin and carboxyhaemoglobin.

Many blood gas analysers, particularly those in emergency departments, are equipped with a channel to measure carboxyhaemoglobin directly

('CO-oximetry'). The haemoglobin of non-smokers may be comprised of up to 3% carboxyhaemoglobin, but this may be as high as 15% in smokers. Levels higher than this are consistent with CO poisoning.

CLINICAL PEARLS

- In order for an observer to detect central cyanosis clinically, received wisdom is that there must be 5 g/dL of reduced haemoglobin, equating to a S_aO_2 of 67% (if Hb is 15 g/dL). This makes cyanosis a late and unreliable sign of hypoxaemia.
- A pulse oximeter may provide a valuable means of home-assessment for patients with long-term respiratory disease, particularly those undergoing long-term non-invasive ventilation. A significant and sustained drop in saturation may provide forewarning of acute deterioration.
- A significant reduction in arterial Po_2 produces only a minimal reduction in oxygen saturation until the steeper part of the oxygen dissociation curve is reached, i.e. a Po_2 of below 10 kPa or a saturation of 94%. Haemoglobin saturation is therefore a less sensitive measure of oxygenation than arterial Po_2, and reliance upon it may miss clinically significant hypoxaemia.
- In a hyperbaric chamber, a patient may breathe 100% oxygen at 3 atm. Under these conditions, the concentration of oxygen in physical solution rises to 6 mL/dL. This alone is sufficient to meet the metabolic needs of the tissues, so that venous blood returns to the heart fully saturated. This hyperoxic environment is toxic to anaerobic bacteria and may be used to treat necrotising soft-tissue infections.

KEY POINTS/SUMMARY

- Pulse oximetry is a non-invasive and completely safe first-line measurement in the breathless patient.
- Readings made by pulse oximetry may differ somewhat from the gold standard measurement of S_aO_2, made on arterial blood.
- Haemoglobin saturation is a factor which determines the arterial oxygen content and, therefore, oxygen delivery to the tissues.
- Haemoglobin saturation gives no information regarding Pco_2 nor ventilation.

12

Assessment of oxygenation

INTRODUCTION

Measurement of oxygenation is a crucial assessment in medicine. Assessment of arterial oxygenation evaluates the overall integrity of pulmonary gas exchange, rather than looking at the constituent processes such as the muscle pump, airway function, and gas transfer, as are measured by conventional lung function. Key measurement parameters are shown in Table 12.1.

NORMAL VALUES

- P_aO_2 – Between 10.6 kPa in the elderly and 13.3 kPa in the young.
- Respiratory failure is defined by an arterial PO_2 <8 kPa.

MEASUREMENT OF P_aO_2

P_aO_2 is traditionally measured by the analysis of a sample of arterial blood, taken from a superficial site such as the radial artery. The composition of arterial blood is the same throughout the systemic circulation. This procedure is relatively safe but somewhat painful. Local anaesthetic may be applied, but this is not routinely employed.

The principle risks of arterial puncture are infection, local nerve injury, and post-puncture bleeding with haematoma, which may compromise the vessel. The risk of the last is particularly increased in those taking anticoagulants, especially if in conjunction with aspirin. For a subject taking anticoagulants, the operator should be certain that arterial puncture is fully warranted before proceeding, but this does not constitute a bar to testing. Arterial puncture should be avoided in severe coagulopathy or following thrombolysis.

Around 1% of the population have no ulnar artery, so that circulation of the hand relies solely upon the radial artery. This may be assessed quickly using Allen's test, which should always be performed prior to arterial

Table 12.1 Key measurement indices/definitions

Parameter	Definition
P_{O_2}	Partial pressure of oxygen in atmospheric air
P_AO_2	Partial pressure of oxygen in alveolar gas
P_aO_2	Partial pressure of oxygen in arterial blood
Arterialised P_{O_2}	Partial pressure of oxygen in arterialised capillary blood

puncture. Absence of collateral circulation by the ulnar artery is a contra-indication to puncture of the radial artery, lest the vessel be damaged. After completion of the procedure, pressure should be applied with a sterile gauze, which should be continued for 5–10 minutes in those who are anticoagulated. Prior to the procedure, patients should be advised of the risks and consent should be sought.

Samples are usually collected in a heparinised tube to delay coagulation and should be analysed at the earliest opportunity for the most accurate results. They should be kept on ice if there is to be any delay in analysis or transportation to the lab.

MEASUREMENT OF ARTERIALISED CAPILLARY P_{O_2}

Sampling of capillary blood provides a less invasive means of oxygenation assessment, which is increasingly employed, particularly in an outpatient or domiciliary setting.[42] Less training is required for healthcare professionals in order to perform this procedure than for arterial puncture. The procedure is better tolerated and complications are likely to be fewer, though they have not been studied.

Capillary blood differs from arterial blood, in partial pressures of both CO_2 and O_2, but particularly the latter which may be up to 8 kPa less than arterial P_{O_2} at rest. However, by applying topical vasodilator (e.g. 'Transvasin'), perfusion of the tissue may be increased to the extent that the local capillary blood becomes 'arterialised' and the blood gas content approximates that of arterial blood. Either the finger or the earlobe has been used for sampling, though blood from the latter is closer in composition to arterial and should be preferred.

The difference in oxygenation between arterial and arterialised capillary specimens has been examined in numerous studies, including a meta-analysis.[43] P_{O_2}

in arterialised capillary blood is on average 0.3 kPa lower than that of arterial blood, with 95% confidence intervals between 0.25 and 0.37 kPa.

A common indication for measurement of P_{O_2} is to determine the need for long-term oxygen therapy (LTOT), which is recommended for those whose resting P_{O_2} level is <7.3 kPa. As this measurement is often performed in patients' homes by nursing staff, capillary sampling is often used.

A study which examined this particular application reported that 9/55 patients assessed would have received LTOT inappropriately, if reliance were placed upon the results of arterialised capillary sampling alone.[44]

Nonetheless, capillary sampling is judged to be a reasonable compromise by many oxygen assessment services which operate in a domiciliary setting. Arguably, services involved in this assessment should quality control their results and consider applying an adjustment factor.

THE OXYGEN CASCADE

Oxygen makes a journey from the atmosphere, through the upper airways, alveoli, arterial blood, and capillaries to the mitochondria. In a perfect system, P_{O_2} would remain at 21 kPa (atmospheric pressure) throughout the

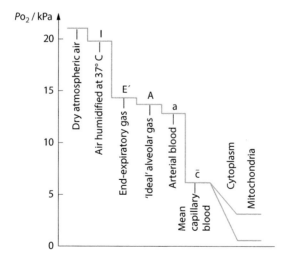

Figure 12.1 The oxygen cascade. (Reprinted from *Nunn's Applied Respiratory Physiology*, 8th edition, Lumb AB, Copyright 2016, with permission from Elsevier.)

system. However, P_{O_2} falls at each successive step of the pathway, creating the 'oxygen cascade' (see Figure 12.1). The existence of a partial pressure gradient from atmospheric air to the mitochondria promotes the net diffusion of oxygen in a one-way direction. Disease at any step may reduce the efficiency of oxygen delivery throughout.

According to Dalton's law, the partial pressure of oxygen in the atmosphere at sea level is equal to the product of barometric pressure (approximately 100 kPa) and the fractional concentration of oxygen (0.21), therefore approximately 21 kPa.

HUMIDIFICATION OF DRY AIR

Inspired air is humidified in the airways by the addition of water vapour, which dilutes the oxygen partial pressure from an atmospheric pressure of 21 kPa to approximately 20 kPa. Therefore, we breathe an effective $F_{I}O_2$ of 0.2.

ALVEOLAR GAS

A significant drop in oxygen tension occurs as inspired air enters the alveoli and mixes with CO_2 found in alveolar gas, which further dilutes the $P_{A}O_2$ to approximately 14 kPa. The factors affecting this value are complex and include altitude/barometric pressure, oxygen consumption, alveolar ventilation, and the respiratory quotient (R). The actual value can be calculated using the alveolar air equation, which is derived elsewhere,[45] but may be represented simply as

$$P_{A}O_2 = P_{I}O_2 - \frac{P_{a}CO_2}{R} \tag{12.1}$$

where $P_{I}O_2$ is the effective partial pressure of oxygen in inspired air. The respiratory quotient depends upon the metabolic substrate, which is determined by the balance of dietary carbohydrate and fat. Typically, R is around 0.8. Therefore, as a rule of thumb

$$P_{A}O_2 = 20 - 1.25 \times P_{a}CO_2 \tag{12.2}$$

Thus, we have an equation that allows easy prediction of alveolar P_{O_2}. Importantly, an understanding of the concept of alveolar P_{O_2} allows calculation of the alveolar–arterial (A–a) P_{O_2} difference, which allows more precise assessment of the efficiency of gas exchange.

Arterial blood

A further drop in partial pressure of oxygen occurs between alveolar gas and the systemic arterial circulation. This step in the oxygen cascade is of great clinical relevance, as the gap between alveolar and arterial P_{O_2} is susceptible to the effects of respiratory disease.

The A–a P_{O_2} difference is calculated by subtracting the calculated P_AO_2 (from Equation 12.1) from the measured P_aO_2 obtained from blood gas analysis.

The A–a P_{O_2} difference should not exceed 2 kPa in healthy young subjects (though it may be higher in healthy elderly subjects).

KEY POINT

The A–a difference provides a means of assessing the expected value of arterial P_{O_2}, taking into account how hard a subject is breathing, as evidenced by the P_{CO_2}.

A–a PARTIAL PRESSURE P_{O_2} DIFFERENCE

Valuable information may be gained about the efficiency of gas exchange by considering the difference between the *measured arterial P_{O_2}* and the *calculated alveolar P_{O_2}* on which it depends. Calculation of the A–a gradient is therefore a powerful tool for evaluation of oxygenation.

Because P_aO_2 depends upon the rate of ventilation, calculation of the A–a gradient allows closer prediction of the expected P_aO_2, *specific to a patient's rate of ventilation*. This is helpful in the following situations, which are illustrated as worked examples.

Example 1

A 25-year-old woman (non-smoker) comes to the emergency department complaining of shortness of breath which started suddenly. She appears anxious. The chest x-ray is normal. She is breathing room air.
Arterial blood gas analysis shows:

$$P_{O_2} = 10.1 \text{ kPa}, \quad P_{CO_2} = 3.7 \text{ kPa}$$

Calculation:
Effective $P_{I_{O_2}}$ is 20 kPa (humidified atmospheric air)

$$\text{Alveolar } P_{O_2} = P_{I_{O_2}} - (1.25 \times P_aCO_2)$$
$$= 20 - 4.5$$
$$= 15.5 \text{ kPa}$$

Alveolar − arterial difference = 15.5 − 10.1
= 5.4 kPa

This woman is therefore significantly hypoxic for her rate of ventilation. That is to say, if she is breathing hard enough to drop her arterial P_{CO_2} to 3.7 kPa, then the arterial P_{O_2} should be much higher. If her A–a gradient were no more than 2 kPa, as may be expected for a woman of her age, then the arterial P_{O_2} would be at least 13.5 kPa. Therefore, a pathological cause of her sudden respiratory compromise should be sought. Possibilities might include asthma (if wheezy) or acute pulmonary embolism.

Example 2

A patient in the emergency department is known to have chronic obstructive pulmonary disease (COPD), having smoked 40/day for 40 years. He presents with shortness of breath increasing over the last few days. He was cyanosed on presentation, so supplemental oxygen was administered (said to be 24%), and arterial blood gases measured:

$$P_{O_2} = 17 \text{ kPa}, P_{CO_2} = 8 \text{ kPa}$$

Calculation:

Effective inspired $P_{I}O_2 = 23$ kPa (humidified)

Calculated alveolar $P_{A}O_2 = P_{I}O_2 − (1.25 \times P_{a}CO_2)$

$$= 23 − (1.25 \times 8)$$

$$= 13 \text{ kPa}$$

Alveolar − arterial difference = 13 − 17
= − 4 kPa (minus 4)

Clearly, this is an impossibility. This combination of P_{CO_2} and P_{O_2} could not arise in a subject breathing an $F_{I}O_2$ of 0.24. Examination of the figures shows that the $F_{I}O_2$ must have been at least 0.3, which would give an A–a gradient of 2 kPa.

24% may have been the *estimated* dose of oxygen, administered using a flow-dependent oxygen mask instead of a Venturi mask. This method is notoriously unreliable and should not be accepted as an alternative to a Venturi mask in patients to whom $F_{I}O_2$ must be carefully regulated.

KEY POINT

As a quick approximation, the sum of arterial P_{O_2} and P_{CO_2} cannot exceed the inspired oxygen concentration.

Example 3

A 70-year-old non-smoker is referred to the respiratory outpatient department with increasing shortness of breath, worse when lying flat. He is fully alert and conscious. Arterial blood gases show:

$$P_{O_2} = 7 \text{ kPa}, P_{CO_2} = 8 \text{ kPa}$$

Clearly the P_{CO_2} is raised, but is oxygenation as good as may be expected?

Calculation:

$$\begin{aligned} \text{Calculated alveolar } P_{O_2} &= P_{O_2} - (1.25 \times P_aCO_2) \\ &= 20 - (1.25 \times 8) \\ &= 10 \text{ kPa} \end{aligned}$$

$$\begin{aligned} \text{Alveolar} - \text{arterial difference} &= 10 - 7 \\ &= 3 \text{ kPa} \end{aligned}$$

The A–a difference is 3 kPa. This is within the expected range for a 70-year-old. This man's gas exchange is normal. The problem here is hypoventilation, as indicated by the raised P_{CO_2}. A neuromuscular cause of diaphragmatic weakness should be suspected, given the history of orthopnoea. No impairment of respiratory gas exchange is suggested by these blood gases.

KEY POINT

Calculation of the A–a P_{O_2} difference is helpful in estimating the predicted arterial P_{O_2} in various scenarios:
- To unmask subtle impairments in gas exchange not otherwise clinically evident.
- When a subject is hypo or hyperventilating.

TISSUE

A large drop in P_{O_2} occurs between the capillary blood and mitochondrial blood, though the latter is difficult to measure. A P_{O_2} of approximately 0.3 kPa is required within mitochondria to fuel oxidative phosphorylation, below which anaerobic metabolism supervenes.

RELATIONSHIP BETWEEN ALVEOLAR P_{O_2} AND ARTERIAL P_{CO_2}

Another way of looking at the alveolar air equation is to calculate the minimum 'expected' arterial P_{O_2} for a given arterial P_{CO_2}, assuming a normal A–a difference. For example, in the case of a 30-year old in good health, we may assume that the A–a difference is no more than 2 kPa.

Starting from Equation (12.2):

$$P_A O_2 = 20 - 1.25 \times P_a CO_2$$

If the A–a difference is 2 kPa, then:

$$P_A O_2 - P_a O_2 = 2$$

Re-arranging:

$$P_A O_2 = P_a O_2 + 2$$

Substituting for $P_A O_2$ in Equation (12.2):

$$P_a O_2 + 2 = 20 - 1.25 \times P_a CO_2$$

$$P_a O_2 = 18 - 1.25 \times P_a CO_2 \tag{12.3}$$

This equation indicates the minimum arterial P_{O_2} expected, based upon an A–a difference of 2 kPa.

Importantly, from Equation (12.3), the relationship between $P_a O_2$ and $P_a CO_2$ may be understood. Several important observations can be made highlighted in the Keypoints below.

KEY POINTS

- Arterial P_{O_2} and P_{CO_2} are inversely related, so that any reduction in one must be associated with an increase in the other (as long as F_iO_2 and R remain constant).
- A patient with mild hypoxia may therefore normalise P_aO_2 by increasing ventilation, thereby reducing P_ACO_2 by 1–2 kPa, bringing a commensurate increase in P_aO_2.

CLINICAL PEARLS

- The highest P_aO_2 attainable breathing room air is constrained by the minimum achievable P_{CO_2}. The lowest values of arterial P_{CO_2} recorded are around 1.7 kPa, which may be reached in high-altitude mountaineers, who ventilate very large minute volumes to compensate for the low atmospheric P_{O_2} at such elevations.
- Likewise, the hyperventilation seen in extreme panic may induce profound hypocapnia. In this high-ventilation state, alveolar P_{O_2} may reach 17–18 kPa. Because there is always a gradient between alveolar and arterial P_{O_2}, arterial P_{O_2} is limited to around 16 kPa.
- By contrast, the maximum arterial P_{CO_2} that may be reached whilst breathing room air is determined by the limit of a patient's tolerance of hypoxaemia. If the arterial P_{O_2} drops as low as 4 kPa, then arterial P_{CO_2} may climb as high as 12 kPa. Consciousness is lost in normal subjects if arterial P_{O_2} drops below about 3.5 kPa, but in chronically hypoxic patients or acclimatised mountaineers, lower values approaching 2.5 kPa may be tolerated.

SPECIFIC CLINICAL CONSIDERATIONS

HYPOXAEMIA

In general physiological terms, there are four causes of arterial hypoxaemia:

- Hypoventilation
- Diffusion limitation
- Shunt (venous admixture)
- Ventilation–perfusion inequality

Under conditions of hypoventilation alveolar P_{CO_2} rises, which dilutes the fractional concentration of oxygen in the alveolar gas. Consequently, arterial P_{O_2} drops.

Ventilation–perfusion mismatch may cause hypoxia if perfusion of underventilated alveoli occurs. This is the most important cause of hypoxia in clinical disease of the lungs. Importantly, each red blood cell passes through only two or three alveoli en route through the lungs and has very limited opportunity to achieve full oxygenation. If a proportion of pulmonary blood flow is directed to a lobe of the lung which is completely consolidated and airless, then this blood will return to the left atrium hypoxaemic and will dilute the saturated haemoglobin within the remaining blood pool.

Diffusion limitation is less common than might be supposed as a cause of hypoxia. Nonetheless, diffusion limitation contributes to hypoxaemia in cases of fibrotic lung disease or pulmonary vasculopathy where the blood–gas barrier becomes thickened.

Shunt (venous admixture) refers to blood which enters the pulmonary veins without traversing ventilated areas of the lung. In normal healthy subjects, a small shunt arises from the bronchial artery and Thebesian coronary vein blood which returns to the systemic circulation without taking part in pulmonary gas exchange. Therefore, in a healthy lung, shunt is responsible for most of the A–a P_{O_2} difference, which does not normally exceed 2 kPa. In conditions of disease, other sources of shunt include abnormal pulmonary arteriovenous fistulae and cardiac septal defects.

APNOEIC RESPIRATION

If a patient becomes apnoeic after a period of breathing 100% oxygen, there is adequate oxygen within the functional residual capacity of the lungs to maintain oxygenation for a considerable period. Furthermore, If airway patency is maintained in an oxygen-rich environment, alveolar oxygenation may be maintained for up to 1 hour, in the absence of breathing.

However, as no ventilation is occuring, alveolar P_{CO_2} rises at a rate of 0.4–0.8 kPa/min, and accumulation of CO_2 within alveoli eventually dilutes the oxygen so that alveolar P_{O_2} falls.

An exercise which illustrates this is undertaken when establishing a diagnosis of brainstem death in ventilated patients, in the setting of severe brain injury. In this protocol, the patient is pre-oxygenated, after which mechanical ventilation is stopped, allowing arterial P_{CO_2} to rise to 6.65 kPa (confirmed by arterial blood gas testing). Failure of any ventilatory response to hypercapnia is one of the criteria required to establish brainstem death. Hypoxia does not occur providing pre-oxygenation was adequate. Moreover, deleterious hypercapnia would ensue before a patient became hypoxic under these circumstances.

CHRONIC RESPIRATORY FAILURE

Assessment for domiciliary long term oxygen therapy (LTOT) is a frequent indication for measuring P_{O_2}. Referral for oxygen assessment is recommended for patients with S_pO_2 <92%.[42]

P_{O_2} is chosen in preference to So_2 as the definitive measure of oxygenation for this purpose, due to the flatness of the oxyhaemoglobin dissociation curve over the range 8–13 kPa. Over this range, a significant change in P_{O_2} may cause little change in So_2, which would make it an imprecise measure.

LTOT therapy has been shown to confer survival benefit for patients with COPD whose arterial P_{O_2} is <7.3 kPa, measured when convalescent – at least 3 weeks after any acute exacerbation (under which circumstances an unrepresentative low reading may occur).

KEY POINTS/SUMMARY

- Respiratory failure exists when arterial P_{O_2} falls below 8 kPa.
- Hypoventilation always causes hypoxaemia and hypercapnia due to the inverse relationship between the two. Mild hypoxaemia may be corrected by increasing ventilation.
- Ventilation–perfusion inequality is the main cause of arterial hypoxaemia, and NOT diffusion limitation as may be intuitively assumed.

13

Assessment of acid–base balance

INTRODUCTION

Metabolism is an oxidative process, the products of which are acidic, including carbon dioxide, lactic acid and citric acid. Acid–base balance is maintained by pulmonary elimination of carbon dioxide and renal excretion of non-volatile acids. A detailed discussion of acid–base biochemistry is beyond the scope of this text, but a method of blood gas data interpretation is presented, with the emphasis on respiratory aspects. The reader is referred to excellent online references for more detailed discussion of this complex area.[46,47]

MEASURED INDICES/KEY DEFINITIONS

The following information may be reported on blood gas analysis, in addition to arterial P_{O_2} and P_{CO_2}. Normal values tend to be supplied by the manufacturers of blood gas analysers, rather than agreed by international consensus. The values given below are in common usage.

pH – The negative log of the hydrogen ion concentration: the more acidic a solution becomes, the lower its pH. The normal range is 7.35–7.45.

The base excess and bicarbonate are calculated from the pH and P_{CO_2}, and so give another way of looking at the same information (see below).

HCO_3^- – The arterial blood bicarbonate concentration, sometimes called actual bicarbonate to distinguish from the standard bicarbonate (below). The normal range is 21–28 mmol/L.

Standard bicarbonate – The concentration of bicarbonate in blood which has been equilibrated with a gas mixture in which the P_{CO_2} is 5.3 kPa (40 mmHg). This is a method of expressing the metabolic component of a disorder, if there were no respiratory compensation. It is the standard bicarbonate rather than the actual bicarbonate which is usually reported on blood gas analysers, though both may be available. The normal range is

> **KEY POINT**
>
> An abnormal standard bicarbonate or base excess indicates a metabolic contribution to an acidosis or alkalosis, but does not indicate whether this is the primary disorder, part of a mixed disturbance, or related to normal physiological compensation.

22–27 mmol/L, with lower values associated with metabolic acidosis and higher values in alkalosis.

Base excess/deficit – The base excess is the quantity of base or acid needed to titrate 1 L of blood to pH 7.4, with the P_{CO_2} held constant at 5.3 kPa. This is another way of quantifying the metabolic component of a derangement. The normal range is ±3 mmol/L, with more negative values found in metabolic acidosis and more positive values in metabolic alkalosis.

PHYSIOLOGY OF ACID–BASE BALANCE

CO_2 is a universal product of metabolism and combines with water to form carbonic acid:

$$CO_2 + H_2O \underset{1}{\overset{(CA)}{\rightleftharpoons}} H_2CO_3 \underset{2}{\rightleftharpoons} H^+ + HCO_3^-$$

The hydration reaction (1) is slow unless catalysed by the enzyme carbonic anhydrase (CA). Despite catalysis, the equilibrium lies far to the left. Carbonic acid (H_2CO_3) formed from this hydration dissociates (2) into its conjugate base (bicarbonate, HCO_3^-) and the hydrogen ion (H^+). A weak acid such as carbonic is largely undissociated, so that the equilibrium of (2) also lies far to the left.

The acidity of the blood is reflected by the ratio of $HCO_3^- : CO_2$ in solution. The normal pH of 7.40 is maintained with a ratio of $HCO_3^- : CO_2$ of 20:1. This is expressed in the Henderson–Hasselbalch equation, the derivation of which may be found elsewhere[46]:

$$pH = 6.1 + \log \frac{\left[HCO_3^- \right]}{0.03 P_{CO_2}}$$

where 6.1 is the pKa (negative logarithm of the acid dissociation constant) for carbonic acid (H_2CO_3) and 0.03 is a factor which relates P_{CO_2} to the amount of CO_2 dissolved in plasma.

If either the P_{CO_2} or the concentration of HCO_3^- alters, physiological compensation involves adjustment of the other parameter, so preserving the ratio and maintaining pH.

COMPENSATION

The respiratory response to metabolic acidosis or alkalosis is mediated by chemosensitive neurones in the brainstem medulla, which are stimulated under conditions of low pH within the cerebrospinal fluid (CSF). These neurones mediate an increase in both the depth and rate of breathing, causing a compensatory change in P_{CO_2}, thereby acting to restore physiological pH.

Likewise, under conditions of respiratory acidosis, the kidneys increase excretion of the acid load. Free H^+ ions cannot be excreted in isolation, so this is achieved by buffering of urinary H^+ by combination with weak acids (titratable acidity). The major titratable acid buffer in urine is phosphate, though this system is not amenable to regulation by the kidney. However, the proximal renal tubules are able to up-regulate metabolism of glutamine to form ammonium (NH_4^+), which is secreted as ammonia (NH_3) into the collecting ducts where it combines with H^+, increasing excretion of the acid load.

KEY POINTS

- Compensation mitigates a derangement of pH by matching an abnormal CO_2 with an abnormal HCO_3^-, (or vice versa) to restore a normal ratio of the two. *Normality* may only be regained by correction of the underlying imbalance.
- Compensation is usually partial rather than total, particularly in the case of respiratory compensation for a metabolic disorder, i.e. pH returns *towards* the normal physiological value, but does not usually reach the normal value.

CLASSIFICATION OF ACID–BASE DISORDERS

The following (slightly confusing) terms are defined:

Acidaemia	pH <7.35
Acidosis	A process which tends to reduce pH, but may be compensated to the extent that pH is within the normal range at the time of measurement.
Alkalaemia	pH >7.45
Alkalosis	A process which tends to raise pH, but may be compensated to the extent that the pH is within the normal range at the time of measurement.

In common usage, the term acidosis is generally applied to any acidotic state, whether compensated or not. Likewise alkalosis. The terms acidaemia and alkalaemia specifically refer to situations where there is pH derangement, but are less commonly used in clinical practice and will not be used in the remainder of this text.

RESPIRATORY DISORDER

In respiratory disorders, derangement of P_{CO_2} is the primary abnormality. Carbon dioxide is an acidic gas, so that any alteration of P_{CO_2} outside the normal range will tend to change the pH, unless compensated.

Respiratory acidosis is seen in any cause of ventilatory failure, due to the effects of CO_2 retention (see 'Causes of hypercapnia' in Chapter 10). Respiratory alkalosis may be seen in response to hypoxia or any other cause of hyperventilation (see 'Causes of low P_{CO_2}' in Chapter 10).

METABOLIC DISORDER

Metabolic acidosis is caused by addition of an acid other than CO_2 to body fluid (usually lactic acid, ketones or uraemic metabolites), or by excessive loss of bicarbonate. In either scenario, HCO_3^- is reduced. The respiratory system compensates by increasing ventilation and eliminating CO_2 in an attempt to restore the HCO_3^-/CO_2 ratio. Common causes are listed in Table 13.1.

Table 13.1 Causes of metabolic acidosis

Increased anion gap	Endogenous acids	Ketoacidosis
		Lactic acidosis
		Uraemia
	Exogenous/poisoning	Methanol
		Ethylene glycol
		Aspirin
Normal anion gap	Loss of bicarbonate	Diarrhoea
		Type 2 (proximal) renal tubular acidosis (RTA)
		Carbonic anhydrase inhibitors
		Ureteric diversion
	Decreased renal acid excretion	Type 1 (distal) RTA

The pathogenesis of metabolic alkalosis is somewhat complex, but is generally linked to loss of strong ions, particularly hypokalaemia. Causes include diuretics, large volume diarrhoea, intestinal villous adenoma, laxative abuse, and mineralocorticoid excess.

EVALUATING COMPENSATION OF ACID–BASE DISTURBANCE

Compensation mitigates a derangement of pH by matching an abnormal CO_2 with an abnormal HCO_3^- (or vice versa) to restore a normal ratio of the two. It is helpful to quantify the degree of compensation which has occurred, for two reasons.

First, understanding the extent of compensation gives some understanding of the chronicity, particularly of a respiratory acidosis. Second, failure to compensate may imply a coexisting derangement. For example, a respiratory acidosis which persists in an uncompensated state may imply a coexisting metabolic acidosis.

There are two approaches to analysis of the relative respiratory and metabolic contributions to a disorder.

The first is simply to look at the base excess and standard bicarbonate. These derived parameters provide a simple expression of the metabolic derangement. A low standard bicarbonate or negative base excess quantify the metabolic contribution of an acidosis. However, use of these parameters does not distinguish between a primary metabolic disorder and the metabolic contribution of a respiratory disorder.[46]

The second, more robust approach is to look at the relationship between the P_{CO_2} and bicarbonate, as below. It is important to use the actual bicarbonate, rather than the standard bicarbonate for these analyses.

Respiratory compensation for metabolic disorder

Respiratory compensation for metabolic acidosis causes the arterial P_{CO_2} to fall approximately by 0.16 kPa for every mmol/L reduction in the serum HCO_3^- concentration.

There is a limit to the scope for respiratory compensation. Even under conditions of severe metabolic acidosis (e.g. serum HCO_3^- concentration <6 mmol/L), the P_{CO_2} is constrained to remain above 1.5 kPa. To achieve such drastic reduction in P_{CO_2}, the minute volume of ventilation may be increased by up to 30 L/min. The duration that such compensation can be maintained is limited by respiratory muscle fatigue.

Likewise, arterial P_{CO_2} does not rise to >7.5 kPa in mitigation of a metabolic alkalosis.

Metabolic compensation for respiratory disorder

Metabolic compensation for acute respiratory acidosis may bring about an increase in HCO_3^- concentration of approximately 0.75 mmol/L for every kPa of abnormal elevation of the P_{CO_2}.

Patients with chronic respiratory acidosis may achieve a greater compensatory rise in serum HCO_3^-, of up to 3.75 mmol/L per kPa elevation in P_{CO_2}. Such a rise may be sufficient to maintain pH in the low-normal range, despite significant chronic elevation of P_{CO_2} to >9 kPa, for example in chronic hypercapnia in patients with stable chronic obstructive pulmonary disease (COPD).

TIME COURSE OF COMPENSATION

Respiratory compensation for metabolic acidosis begins within 30 minutes and is complete within 12–24 hours. Therefore, if a metabolic acidosis develops gradually, respiratory compensation may keep pace so that severe acidosis never occurs.

Metabolic compensation for respiratory acidosis occurs in two stages. There is an immediate, small change in serum HCO_3^- (in the same direction as the PCO_2 change), which is due to intracellular buffering of CO_2 by phosphate and cellular proteins, particularly haemoglobin in erythrocytes.

If the respiratory disorder persists for more than minutes to hours, then renal compensation supervenes, which takes 3–5 days for completion.

SUMMARY: EVALUATION OF ACID–BASE DISORDERS

The changes are summarised in Table 13.2.

1. First, look at the pH. Is there an acidosis or alkalosis?
2. Look at the arterial PCO_2; this indicates the origin of the disorder. If the arterial PCO_2 is raised, an acidosis is of respiratory origin, if low or normal it is metabolic.

If the pH is normal despite a raised PCO_2, then there is a fully compensated respiratory acidosis. This must be chronic in duration.

Table 13.2 Changes in blood gas parameters occurring in respiratory failure

	PO_2 (kPa)	PCO_2 (kPa)	pH	HCO_3^- (mM)	BE (mM)
Normal	>10.6	<6.5	7.35–7.45	21–28	±3
Type 1	↓	↓/↔	↔	↔	↔
Type 2 acute	↓	↑	↓	↔	↔
Type 2 chronic	↓	↑	↔	↑	↑
Type 2 acute on chronic	↓	↑↑	↓	↑	↑

3. Is there appropriate compensation for the disorder? Is the change in bicarbonate commensurate with the change on P_{CO_2} in the case of respiratory disorder (or vice versa)? In the case of respiratory acidosis, is this acute or chronic?

If compensation has not occurred as expected, then there may be a mixed respiratory/metabolic disorder.

KEY POINTS/SUMMARY

- The P_{CO_2} indicates the origin of an acid–base disorder.
- Respiratory acidosis may be fully compensated by an increase in renal elimination of NH_4^+.
- Metabolic acidosis or alkalosis may be partially compensated by respiratory adjustments of arterial P_{CO_2}.

PART 3

EXERCISE TESTING

14

Field exercise tests

INTRODUCTION

Field exercise tests are simple performance measures of endurance or maximal capacity, which may be performed at remote sites without reliance upon lab facilities. Whilst not specifically tests of pulmonary function, these tests assess global functional status, of which the respiratory system is a vital component. The advantages offered by exercise testing are several-fold:

- Subtle impairment of pulmonary functional status may be unmasked by exercise, before it is evident on resting lung function.
- The quantification of functional status is useful in the assessment of response to various clinical interventions such as pulmonary rehabilitation, bronchodilator therapy and the efficacy of ambulatory oxygen.
- Field exercise tests provide prognostic information, including mortality prediction.
- If oxyhaemoglobin desaturation occurs during exercise, then respiratory disease is implicated as a cause of exercise limitation.
- Field exercise tests have an important role in determining fitness for major surgery.

MEASUREMENT INDICES

The primary measurements made during field exercise tests are the distance walked (metres), arterial oxygen saturation (S_pO_2), and the endurance time (minutes).

These simple indices give a surprisingly large amount of information regarding functional status, prognosis, and causation of any exercise intolerance. Furthermore, a record of perceived exertion, given by an index such as the Borg rating of perceived exertion (RPE), can offer an indication of a patient's own perception of exercise intensity and/or breathlessness, which may be useful in combination with physiological measurements to confirm a good volitional effort.

DESCRIPTION OF TESTS

A variety of field exercise tests exist, which range in terms of simplicity, equipment required, and measurements made. These include the following:

6-minute walk test (6MWT)
Incremental shuttle walk test (ISWT)
Endurance shuttle walk test (ESWT)

Field exercise tests are simple to perform, require little comprehension, and may be accomplished by most subjects. Exhaustive lists of exercise test contraindications are available,[48] but notably unstable cardiovascular status or a myocardial infarction within 3 weeks, a resting tachycardia above 120 bpm, or resting hypertension (systolic blood pressure >180 mmHg or diastolic blood pressure >100 mmHg) all warrant caution.

If worrying symptoms develop during testing then the procedure should be terminated. Most of these are obvious, but include chest pain, sweating, pallor, unsteadiness of gait or dizziness.

SIX-MINUTE WALK TEST

The most commonly performed field exercise test is the 6MWT or 6-minute walk distance (6MWD) test.

The test is performed between two cones over a course which should be as long as possible, preferably about 30 m. Shorter courses have been found to produce shorter walking distances. The patient walks back and forth around cones as many times as possible in 6 minutes. The walking speed is self-paced, although in the patient briefing the need to walk the furthest distance possible should be emphasised. The patient may slow down or even stop to rest, but should understand the need to resume walking as soon as possible.

Importantly, the patient should receive only standardised information and encouragement during the walk, as the 6MWD is very sensitive to variation in methodology, including encouragement. No minimum S_pO_2 has been standardised for test termination, though some protocols instruct termination in the event of S_pO_2 <80% and such protocols have an excellent safety record. Well-being should be assessed by a combination of patient symptoms and appearance as well as S_pO_2.

The distance walked (6MWD) is the primary outcome measure, but the minimum saturation value recorded is also an important marker of disease severity and prognosis. At the end of the 6 minutes, recovery should be monitored until resting heart rate, S_pO_2, and Borg rating approach resting measurements.

INCREMENTAL SHUTTLE WALK TEST

The test is performed between two cones 9 m apart to the accompaniment of a series of bleeps, which are sounded at progressively shorter intervals. The subject walks back and forth around the cones, reaching the next cone by the time the next bleep occurs.

The test is terminated when the subject is unable to match the pace of the bleeps or in the event of worrisome symptoms as above. At the end of the test distance, heart rate, S_pO_2, and Borg scale are recorded, as well as the reason for test termination.

ENDURANCE SHUTTLE WALK TEST

The ESWT appears exactly the same as the ISWT, except that the pace of the timing bleeps remains constant throughout the test. This test is usually performed after an ISWT, which allows selection of an appropriate pace approximating 85% of the patient's peak. The greatest utility of the ESWT is to provide a standardised comparison of functional status before and after interventional strategies.

CHOICE OF FIELD-WALKING TEST

All walking tests provide strong prognostic and survival stratification for patients with chronic respiratory disease, more so for patients with chronic obstructive pulmonary disease (COPD) than for interstitial lung disease (ILD). There is a lack of evidence to show superiority of one test over another.

The ISWT is an incremental test of maximal capacity, whereas the 6MWT provides a better reflection of everyday activity. The ISWT is externally paced, whereas the 6MWT is self-paced. Nonetheless, both may be associated with similar oxygen consumption ($\dot{V}_{O_2}$) to that attained during a maximal cardiopulmonary exercise test protocol[48] (see Chapter 15).

The 6MWT is the most commonly employed test due to its convenience, minimal equipment requirement, and reasonable standardisation. This test remains popular for pre-operative functional assessments and disability evaluation. The 6MWT may be criticised for overestimating disability due to the self-paced nature of the test and risk of submaximal effort or pace.

The ESWT, if performed at an appropriate pace, is more sensitive to successful interventions such as pulmonary rehabilitation or bronchodilator therapy when used for patients with COPD.

PHYSIOLOGY OF FIELD EXERCISE TESTS

The pulmonary and cardiovascular systems are designed to have large reserves of function for use at times of exercise and increased energy expenditure. These reserves allow for an increase in oxygen supply to working muscles and tissues to match increased energy demands of aerobic metabolism.

The respiratory system does not work at its full capacity in a healthy subject, even at maximal exercise, as cardiovascular constraints are the usual limiting factors. Thus, at maximal exercise, a normal subject has capacity for a voluntary increase in ventilation of the lungs. Furthermore, diffusive flux of respiratory gases should be sufficient to prevent significant arterial oxygen desaturation.

The cardiovascular system also has large reserves, but cardiovascular capacity in a normal individual is more closely correlated to maximal performance; stroke volume, heart rate, and therefore cardiac output should reach their respective maxima at peak exercise levels.

In a disease state, reserves of cardiovascular and pulmonary function may be markedly reduced. Significant airflow limitation will reduce ventilatory capacity, to the point that ventilatory limitation occurs before predicted maximal workload is achieved. Decreased pulmonary compliance due to interstitial lung disease has a similar effect, although breathing patterns will be different (see Chapter 15). All pulmonary disorders will cause ventilation–perfusion mismatch, and ultimately result in arterial oxygen desaturation.

Cardiac disorders do not cause a reduced arterial oxygen saturation, even at maximal exercise, and this represents a fundamental difference between field exercise test results in cardiac and pulmonary disorders.

NORMAL VALUES

S_pO_2 – Normal oxyhaemoglobin saturation is 98% and does not decline appreciably during exercise, with a 4% desaturation an arbitrary limit of normality.

Six-minute walk test

Several attempts have been made to identify a normal walking distance for the 6MWT.

The American Thoracic Society has stated that average 6MWT distances are 580 m for males and 500 m for females.[49]

A subsequent international study reported a mean 6MWD of 571 ± 90 m.[50] Although regression equations were developed, there was significant variability and the use of predictive equations was not recommended.

If the 6MWT is repeated, for example after an intervention, then a change of 30 m is taken as the threshold for a significant change from baseline (minimum important difference [MID]). However, many subjects show a significant learning effect, so that a 6MWD of up to 25 m longer is attained on a second attempt, even in the absence of any intervention. Therefore, there is a case for performing two-baseline 6MWTs prior to any intervention, of which the value from the better should be recorded.

Incremental shuttle walk test

A reference equation for the ISWT has been developed:[51]

$$ISWT \text{ distance (m)} = 1449.701 - (11.735 \times Age \text{ (yr)}) + (241.897 \times Sex) - (5.686 \times BMI)$$

where Sex = 1 for male and 0 for females.

Endurance shuttle walk test

Reference equations or predicted values have yet to be established for the ESWT. However, a normal minimum distance of >400 m for shuttle walk tests in general has been suggested as a cut-off for good post-operative function following lung cancer surgery. The sensitivity of the ESWT for identifying successful therapeutic interventions has also prompted an MID between pre- and post-intervention ESWT results to be established at 45–85 s or 60–115 m.

CLINICAL PEARLS

An impromptu exercise test may be performed in the clinic area, by walking a patient along the corridor and back whilst monitoring oxygen saturation. Although this test lacks any standardisation, it may provide invaluable information on a subject who complains of significant dyspnoea without a readily apparent cause. Chronic thromboembolic disease is a condition which may cause significant desaturation despite relative preservation of resting lung function.

CHRONIC OBSTRUCTIVE PULMONARY DISEASE

The BODE index is probably the most valuable prognostic tool for assessment of mortality for patients with COPD.[52] The 6MWD is one element of the BODE index (Body mass index [BMI], Obstruction, Dyspnoea and Exercise). A 6MWD of greater than 350 m scores zero in this index and so confers no adverse prognosis (Table 14.1). The modified Medical Research Council (mMRC) scale of breathlessness is shown in Table 14.2.

PULMONARY HYPERTENSION

Dramatic arterial oxygen desaturation is often seen during exercise in those with pulmonary vascular disorders such a primary pulmonary artery

Table 14.1 The BODE index of functional status

	0	1	2	3
$FEV_1\%$ pred	≥65	50–64	36–49	≤35
6MWD (m)	≥350	230–349	150–249	≤149
mMRC	0–1	2	3	4
BMI	>21	≤21		

Table 14.2 The modified MRC dyspnoea scale

Modified MRC dyspnoea scale
0   Breathless only with strenuous exercise.
1   Short of breath when hurrying on the level or walking up a slight hill.
2   Slower than most people of the same age on the level because of breathlessness or have to stop for breath when walking at my own pace on the level.
3   Stop for breath after walking about 100 m or after a few minutes at my own pace on the level.
4   Too breathless to leave the house or I am breathless when dressing.

hypertension (PAH). Destruction of pulmonary capillaries restricts pulmonary blood flow through the capillary bed, creating large ventilation–perfusion inequalities. Consequently, field exercise tests, particularly the 6MWT, are routinely used to monitor disease progression and response to treatment in patients with pulmonary hypertension.

KEY POINTS

- Field exercise tests measure global functional status, which is useful in the assessment of unexplained dyspnoea, response to treatment, disability, disease severity/prognosis and fitness for surgery.
- Reduced walking distance on field exercise tests identifies exercise intolerance, which can be a better indication of mortality prognosis than resting lung function indices.
- Arterial oxygen desaturation is a distinguishing feature of pulmonary disease, be it of the airways, interstitium, or pulmonary vasculature.

15

Cardiopulmonary exercise testing

INTRODUCTION

Cardiopulmonary exercise testing (CPET, CPEX) offers a fully quantifiable measurement of physiological status and maximal aerobic capacity. A full description of this test and its interpretation is beyond the scope of this text but is the subject of many others (see 'Further reading'). As CPET is increasingly employed, a brief consideration of the basic principles is presented.

CPET has a multitude of established applications including determination of fitness for major surgery, investigation of dyspnoea in complex cases, and fitness assessments. Performance-limiting abnormalities of either the respiratory or the cardiovascular systems may be identified.

Moreover, the pattern of results may specifically indicate deconditioning, allowing for a positive diagnosis of a lack of fitness in those whose breathlessness persists despite normal resting investigations. Indeed, robust diagnosis of normality is often the role of CPET in respiratory clinics for those with unexplained exercise intolerance or breathlessness.

MEASURED INDICES/KEY DEFINITIONS

Table 15.1 shows the key parameters which may be calculated from data produced during CPET.

TEST DESCRIPTION/TECHNIQUE

CPET can be undertaken by any individual capable of performing the chosen exercise modality, which may be an exercise cycle ergometer, treadmill, or arm crank. There are several contraindications, which should be carefully considered before subjecting an individual to a maximal exercise test.

Table 15.1 Key parameters derived from cardiopulmonary exercise testing

Index	Abbreviation	Units	Definition and notes
Peak oxygen consumption	$\dot{V}_{O_2PEAK}$	mL/min/kg	The maximum level of oxygen consumption achieved by an individual before exercise is terminated. This is the primary index used to indicate exercise capacity and tolerance. The measurement is usually expressed per body weight. In athletes and well-motivated healthy individuals, this is often termed $\dot{V}_{O_2MAX}$, but $\dot{V}_{O_2PEAK}$ is preferred in clinical practice because exercise may be terminated before a true volitional maximum is achieved by a patient population.
Anaerobic threshold	AT	mL/min/kg	The exercise intensity beyond which anaerobic metabolism is increasingly required to meet energy demand, identified by the oxygen consumption at that point, hence the $\dot{V}_{O_2}$ @ AT.
Peak heart rate	HR_{PEAK}	Beats per minute (bpm)	The maximum HR that an individual can achieve at peak exercise.
Oxygen pulse	$\dot{V}_{O_2}$/HR	mL/HR	The oxygen consumption divided by the HR at any given work rate, giving the oxygen consumption extracted from each heartbeat. As cardiac output is also a product of HR (CO = HR × SV), oxygen pulse is often used as a surrogate of stroke volume.

(Continued)

Table 15.1 (Continued) Key parameters derived from cardiopulmonary exercise testing

Index	Abbreviation	Units	Definition and notes
Ventilatory capacity	$\dot{V}_{Ecap}$ or MVV	L/min	The theoretical maximal minute ventilation that an individual can achieve. This may be extrapolated from the arduous maximal voluntary ventilation (MVV) test, a brief (12–15 s) period of maximal hyperventilation. However, it is more conveniently estimated from FEV_1, usually $35–40 \times FEV_1$, depending on the test population. The $\dot{V}_{Ecap}$ is seldom achieved in health, even at peak exercise, but is an important concept from which the breathing reserve is derived (see below).
Breathing reserve	BR	L/min or %	The difference between peak exercise ventilation and theoretical maximal ventilation ($\dot{V}_{Ecap}$). This can be expressed either in absolute terms or calculated as a percentage from the equation $100\ [\dot{V}_{Ecap} - \text{peak exercise ventilation}]/\dot{V}_{Ecap}$. A reduction in breathing reserve at peak exercise suggests ventilatory limitation to exercise capacity. Lower values occur in both airway and restrictive lung disease, and help to distinguish between cardiovascular and pulmonary causes of exercise intolerance.
Ventilatory equivalent for CO_2	$\dot{V}_E/\dot{V}_{CO_2}$	No units	The ratio of $\dot{V}_E$ to $\dot{V}_{CO_2}$, which represents the rate of ventilation required per unit rate of CO_2 production. In other words, it is an indication of ventilatory efficiency, with lower values representing better efficiency. The value of this parameter is of particular interest at the anaerobic threshold ($\dot{V}_E/\dot{V}_{CO_2}$ @ AT). Alternatively, this value can be displayed graphically as the slope of the relationship between $\dot{V}_E$ and $\dot{V}_{CO_2}$, with a steeper slope representing less efficient ventilation.

(Continued)

Table 15.1 (Continued) Key parameters derived from cardiopulmonary exercise testing

Index	Abbreviation	Units	Definition and notes
Ventilatory equivalent for O_2	$\dot{V}_E/\dot{V}_{O_2}$	No units	The ratio of $\dot{V}_E$ to $\dot{V}_{O_2}$, analogous to above. Changes to this parameter in relation to the changes in $\dot{V}_E/\dot{V}_{CO_2}$ (above) can be used to help identify the anaerobic threshold during incremental exercise testing.
Respiratory exchange ratio	RER	No units	The ratio of $\dot{V}_{CO_2}$ to $\dot{V}_{O_2}$. This value changes with diet (due to the available energy substrate). The value of the RER also rises with exercise intensity.
$\dot{V}_{O_2}$/heart rate relationship	$\dot{V}_{O_2}$/HR	mL/beat	The slope of the graph of oxygen consumption against HR during an incremental exercise test.
$\dot{V}_{O_2}$/work rate relationship	$\Delta\dot{V}_{O_2}/\Delta WR$	mL/min/W	The slope of the relationship between $\dot{V}_{O_2}$ and work rate during an incremental exercise test. Low values may indicate a reduction in peripheral oxygen delivery.

Most of these involve unstable cardiovascular or respiratory status to avoid precipitating an acute event.

The most commonly employed CPET protocol employs a progressively incremental workload which continues until exercise cannot be sustained or physiological parameters necessitate exercise termination. For most reliable results, the incremental exercise period should last between 8 and 12 minutes. The rate of workload increase is selected according to the predicted $\dot{V}_{O_2PEAK}$, age, gender and habitual levels of activity of the subject.

The exercise modality may influence results, with treadmill exercise usually producing greater $\dot{V}_{O_2PEAK}$ values. However, cycle ergometers may offer other benefits in terms of space, convenience, safety, and consistency of test results.

PHYSIOLOGY OF EXERCISE TESTING

Maximal exercise is normally limited by the ability of the cardiovascular system to deliver oxygenated blood to the working muscles, despite the capacity for cardiac output to increase by many multiples of basal resting activity. Cardiovascular constraints are such that healthy individuals are not normally able to reach the limits of their respiratory system reserve, neither in terms of ventilation nor gas diffusing capacity.

Characteristic patterns of abnormality may reveal which system is responsible for reduced exercise tolerance, and in some cases identify the cause of any pathology that may exist.

Normal physiological responses

Under conditions of maximal exercise, cardiac output rises from its resting rate of 5 L/min to a maximum of around 20 L/min. Initially, the increase in cardiac output is achieved by an increase in both heart rate (HR) and stroke volume, with stroke volume increasing from 80 to about 110 mL. Thereafter, any further increase in cardiac output is achieved primarily by increasing the HR.

Systemic systolic blood pressure rises from 120 mmHg at rest to values of 200–250 mmHg. By contrast, diastolic blood pressure normally increases by 10–15 mmHg or less.

Ventilation also increases from its resting rate of 5–10 L/min to around 200 L/min in a conditioned subject. At low and moderate workloads, the increase is accommodated by increasing tidal volume up to approximately 65% of vital capacity. Beyond this, further demand is met by increasing respiratory rate up to a normal maximum of around 55 breaths/min.

Despite substantial cardiorespiratory reserve as above, these increases are insufficient to fully meet the demands of high-intensity exercise. Further capacity is provided by extraction of a greater proportion of the blood oxygen content than occurs under resting conditions. Thus, a greater arteriovenous oxygen difference (a-vo_2 difference) develops.

As exercise intensity increases, even this additional capacity is exceeded and to keep pace any further energy requirement must be met by anaerobic metabolism. This results in the production of lactate as a byproduct of anaerobic glycolysis.

Buffering of this lactate in the blood provides an additional CO_2 load. Therefore, as anaerobic metabolism increases, the rate of CO_2 elimination rises in relation to the rate of oxygen utilisation. The point at which this occurs is termed the anaerobic threshold (or lactate threshold), and is signified by a change in the slope of the $\dot{V}_{CO_2}/\dot{V}_{O_2}$ graph (see Figure 15.1).

As exercise approaches its highest intensity, the buffering capacity of the blood becomes exhausted, so that acidosis occurs. This creates an additional stimulation to ventilation, which results in a physiological hyperventilation. At this stage,

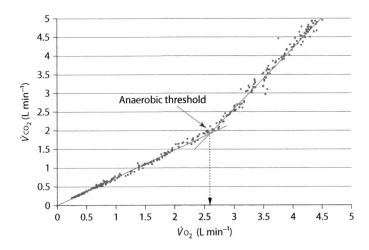

Figure 15.1 Anaerobic threshold (AT). The identification of the AT via the 'V-slope' method, showing the change in relationship between $\dot{V}_{O_2}$ and $\dot{V}_{CO_2}$ as reliance on anaerobic metabolism increases at more intensive workloads.

termed the respiratory compensation (RC) point, the level of ventilation becomes uncoupled from its usual tightly regulated relationship with the rate of CO_2 production. Exercise is not usually sustainable at this level of intensity.

Expired respiratory gas concentrations are measured during CPET. Oxygen consumption is a direct index of the work being done. The work level attained at maximal exercise is termed $\dot{V}_{O_2 PEAK}$ or $\dot{V}_{O_2 MAX}$ if certain stringent criteria are met which define true maximal output. $\dot{V}_{O_2}$ increases from approximately 250 mL/min at rest to about 4 L/min in trained subjects at peak exercise.

The normal patterns of response for the major physiological parameters measured during CPET are as follows:

- *HR*: Shows a linear increase during incremental exercise (Figure 15.2).
- *Ventilation*: Increases in a curvilinear fashion during incremental exercise (Figure 15.3).
- $\dot{V}_{O_2}$: Shows a linear increase during incremental exercise (Figure 15.4).
- $\dot{V}_{CO_2}$: Initially shows a linear increase during incremental exercise, followed by a steeper ascent under conditions of anaerobic metabolism.
- $\Delta\dot{V}_{O_2}/\Delta WR$: Shows a linear relationship during an incremental exercise test.
- *Oxygen pulse*: Increases with exercise intensity, but this increase may slow towards peak exercise intensity (Figure 15.2).

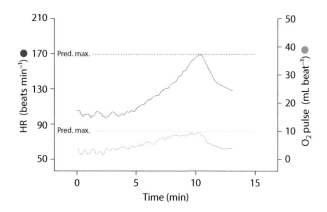

Figure 15.2 Heart rate (HR) and oxygen pulse during incremental exercise. The rise in both HR (darker line) and oxygen pulse (lighter line) over time during an incremental exercise test. Both values increase linearly to their respective peak predicted values at maximal exercise intensity. However, the rate of increase in oxygen pulse may slow towards peak exercise.

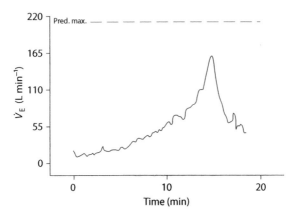

Figure 15.3 Ventilation during incremental exercise. The graph shows the increase in ventilation over time during an incremental exercise test. Ventilation increases in a curvilinear fashion. In normal healthy individuals, ventilation does not reach its predicted maximum, indicating that ventilation is not a normal limiting factor to exercise tolerance.

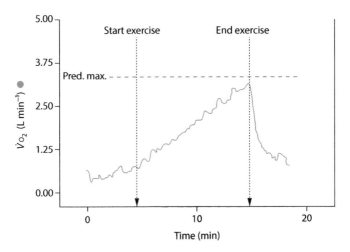

Figure 15.4 Oxygen consumption during incremental exercise. The graph shows the rise in oxygen consumption ($\dot{V}_{O_2}$) over time during an incremental exercise test. Oxygen consumption increases linearly up to its predicted peak.

- $\dot{V}_E/\dot{V}_{CO_2}$: reduces (i.e. improved ventilatory efficiency) up to and just beyond the anaerobic threshold, increasing thereafter until peak exercise intensity (shown in Figure 15.5a). Note that $\dot{V}_E/\dot{V}_{O_2}$ reaches a nadir at the anaerobic threshold, before the nadir in $\dot{V}_E/\dot{V}_{CO_2}$.

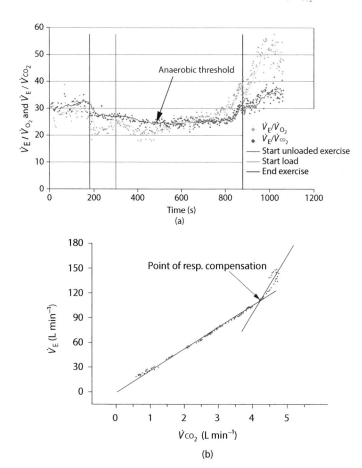

Figure 15.5 Ventilatory efficiency. (a) Time course of ventilatory equivalents for both oxygen ($\dot{V}_E/\dot{V}_{O_2}$) and carbon dioxide ($\dot{V}_E/\dot{V}_{CO_2}$) during an incremental exercise test. Note that the $\dot{V}_E/\dot{V}_{O_2}$ (lighter dots) reaches a nadir at the anaerobic threshold, with the $\dot{V}_E/\dot{V}_{CO_2}$ (darker) reaching a nadir sometime thereafter. (b) Relationship between ventilation and $\dot{V}_{CO_2}$ before and after the point of respiratory compensation.

Further intense exercise beyond the point of RC results in the uncoupling of ventilation and $\dot{V}_{CO_2}$ (see Figure 15.5b).

- *Systemic blood pressure:* Systolic blood pressure increases with exercise intensity, with a smaller increase in diastolic pressure, resulting in a widening of pulse pressure.
- *Electrocardiogram (ECG):* The ECG shows an increase in HR, but should show no development of significant ectopic activity, S-T segment depression (>2.0–2.5 mm), T-wave inversion nor bundle branch block.

NORMAL VALUES

Normal values for the main exercise parameters, either at peak exercise or at the anaerobic threshold, are shown below:

- $\dot{V}_{O_2PEAK}$: A maximal oxygen consumption of greater than 84% of the predicted value, based upon age, height, and gender, is considered normal for sedentary individuals.
- $\Delta\dot{V}_{O_2}/\Delta WR$: The slope of this graph is remarkably consistent in health across all ages, sexes, and physical capabilities at around 10 mL/min/W, with a lower limit of normality of 8.6 mL/min/W.[53]
- $\dot{V}_{O_2}$ @ AT: The anaerobic threshold normally occurs at an oxygen consumption which is greater than 40% of the predicted $\dot{V}_{O_2PEAK}$. Also, a $\dot{V}_{O_2}$ @ AT of >11.0 mL/min/kg is widely used as a cut-off for a favourable prognosis in pre-surgical assessment.[54]
- *Peak HR:* HR should reach a peak value calculated from the following formula:

$$\text{Peak heart rate} = 208 - (0.7 \times \text{age}).$$

This formula is considered more applicable in the majority of situations than the more familiar formula of 220 – age.[55]
- *Peak O_2 pulse:* The oxygen pulse should reach a peak value greater than 80% of the predicted peak value. The rate of increase may slow toward peak exercise, but the oxygen pulse should not decline before the end of the incremental stage of the exercise test.
- *Breathing reserve:* In normal individuals, a breathing reserve of >11 L/min or 15% should remain at peak exercise. A lower value may be seen in highly trained individuals and should be interpreted in context.

- $\dot{V}_E/\dot{V}_{CO_2}$ @ *AT*: Reference equations are available, but a value <35 at the anaerobic threshold is generally considered normal.
- S_pO_2: A desaturation of ≥4% or greater is considered abnormal. Paradoxically, elite athletes may exhibit a desaturation at extreme workloads, but such a finding should be interpreted in context.

PATTERNS OF ABNORMALITY

EXERCISE TOLERANCE

$\dot{V}_{O_2PEAK}$ is the primary index of exercise capacity (Figure 15.4). A reduced value may be due to a variety of causes, including disease, deconditioning, anxiety, or obesity. Abnormal exercise limitation should only be reported if several variables meet predicted maximal values. These include reaching at least 85% of predicted peak HR and a respiratory exchange ratio greater than 1.15. A submaximal test should be suspected if these values are not achieved.

LUNG DISEASE

A reduction in breathing reserve at maximal exercise is the cardinal feature of lung disease, whether obstructive or restrictive in nature.

Limitation of breathing reserve is intuitively understood in cases of obstructive disease, under which circumstances airway disease prevents airflow increasing to match the requirements of energy demand. This is illustrated in Figure 15.6, which shows ventilation at maximal exercise impinging upon the theoretical maximum ventilatory capacity ($\dot{V}_{ECAP}$, see Table 15.1). Peak ventilation may exceed this theoretical maximum due to the bronchodilator effects of endogenous adrenaline released during exercise. However, healthy subjects seldom approach their theoretical $\dot{V}_{ECAP}$, retaining at least 15% breathing reserve at peak exercise. In subjects with dynamic hyperinflation, tidal volume may be seen to decline as breathing reserve diminishes, due to the limitation which airway obstruction poses to exhalation.

Restrictive disease is usually accompanied by an increased respiratory frequency (above 55 breaths/min) at peak exercise, in an attempt to achieve

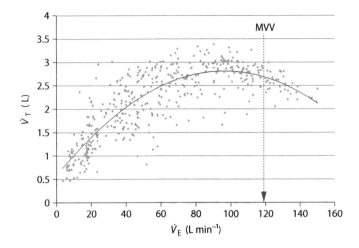

Figure 15.6 Relationship between ventilation and tidal volume during incremental exercise. In this case, Ventilation exceeds the theoretical predicted ventilatory capacity (MVV), indicating an abnormal ventilatory limitation to exercise tolerance. Reduction in tidal volume towards peak exercise levels suggests the occurrence of dynamic hyperinflation in this subject.

adequate ventilation despite pathologically low lung volumes. Inadequate ventilation often persists regardless, causing ventilation–perfusion mismatch, with desaturation and significant reduction in ventilatory efficiency at the anaerobic threshold (increased $\dot{V}_E/\dot{V}_{CO_2}$ @ AT). Inevitably, exercise will be terminated prematurely due to ventilatory limitation, so that HR fails to reach predicted maximal values.

Heart disease – Ischaemic heart disease

By contrast to patients with lung disease, breathing reserve remains normal or high at exercise termination in subjects with ischaemic heart disease because exercise is limited by cardiovascular dysfunction. At the work rate where myocardial ischaemia begins to limit contractility, HR starts to rise at a disproportionately greater rate to $\dot{V}_{O_2}$ (see Figure 15.7). At this point, the $\dot{V}_{O_2}$–HR graph extrapolates back to an intercept approaching or even below zero (as in Figure 15.8), and the oxygen pulse (a surrogate for stroke

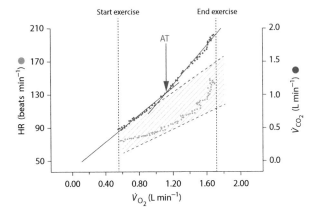

Figure 15.7 HR response during myocardial ischaemia. The lighter plot shows an increase is seen in the HR–$\dot{V}_{O_2}$ slope typical of that seen in subjects with myocardial ischaemia. Ischaemia causes a reduction in myocardial contractility, necessitating a compensatory increase in HR in an attempt to maintain cardiac output. The crossed hatched area represents the normal range of the HR–$\dot{V}_{O_2}$ relationship, but the slope of the response should be linear in health. The darker plot shows the relationship between $\dot{V}_{CO_2}$ and $\dot{V}_{O_2}$, indicating the anaerobic threshold (AT).

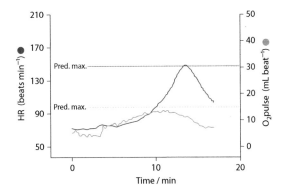

Figure 15.8 Decline in oxygen pulse due to myocardial ischaemia. The oxygen pulse graph (lighter plot) is seen to fall shortly after 10 minutes. Myocardial ischaemia is the most likely explanation for a decline in the oxygen pulse (in the absence of arterial oxygen desaturation or an abnormal widening of the A–a gradient). Ischaemia causes a reduction in myocardial contractility, necessitating a compensatory increase in HR in an attempt to maintain cardiac output. Note that under conditions of ischaemia, the HR is not linear during the incremental phase (compare with Figure 15.2).

volume) plateaus or even declines. This may coincide with ECG S-T segment and/or T-wave changes, a reduction in systolic blood pressure and possibly symptoms of angina.

The oxygen pulse plateaus early because cardiac output is limited or may even decline. A decline in the oxygen pulse, or extrapolation of the $\dot{V}_{O_2}$–HR graph to an intercept below zero, indicates that ventricular contractility may be compromised. If this coincides with a decline in systolic blood pressure of greater that 20 mmHg then exercise termination should be considered. Occasionally, due to changes in cardiac preload and afterload, the oxygen pulse may exhibit a paradoxical increase at exercise termination.

Arterial oxygen saturation remains unchanged, which is key in distinguishing cardiac from pulmonary limitation.

HEART DISEASE – CARDIOMYOPATHY

Patients with heart failure have a high ventilatory requirement at low work rates because poor oxygen delivery leads to relatively early metabolic acidosis, necessitating RC. Therefore, there is reduced ventilatory efficiency (high $\dot{V}_E/\dot{V}_{CO_2}$ @ AT) or a steeper $\dot{V}_E/\dot{V}_{CO_2}$ slope. S_pO_2 remains unchanged. The HR response for any given $\dot{V}_{O_2}$ is steep, and a unique oscillating ventilatory pattern is sometimes seen which may be analogous to sleep-related Cheyne–Stokes respiration. The oxygen pulse may be flat, with low peak values and a paradoxical increase upon exercise termination.

PULMONARY VASCULAR DISEASE

An increase in pulmonary vascular resistance prevents appropriate increase in cardiac output, leading to significant ventilation–perfusion mismatch. Consequently a disproportionately high ventilatory response is required at relatively low workloads, with a flat and unchanging oxygen pulse (see Figure 15.9) and reduced ventilatory efficiency (increased $\dot{V}_E/\dot{V}_{CO_2}$ @ AT). Post-exercise increases in the oxygen pulse are not usually seen, but reductions in S_pO_2 are progressive throughout exercise and often profound. A sudden drop in arterial oxygen saturations towards peak exercise may suggest the presence of an R–L cardiac shunt.

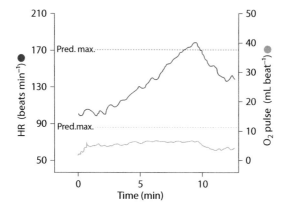

Figure 15.9 Flat oxygen pulse in pulmonary vasculopathy. A flat oxygen pulse plot is characteristically seen during incremental workload exercise tests in patients suffering from pulmonary vascular disorders and pulmonary hypertension. This response is usually accompanied by arterial oxygen desaturation, but a sudden drop in arterial oxygen saturations near to peak exercise may suggest the presence of a co-existing ventricular septal defect and a right-to-left intra-cardiac shunt.

SUMMARY

Table 15.2 summarises physiological responses during and after CPET, although it should be noted that the values chosen are selective and by no means exhaustive. CPET results do not always conform to the expected pattern in real-life tests. $\dot{V}_{O_2\text{PEAK}}$ is not included in this table as it is reduced in all pathological conditions which compromise the cardiovascular or respiratory systems. Variables highlighted in bold have particular discriminative value.

ASSESSMENT OF SEVERITY

CPET evaluations are not ordinarily used for the purposes of grading severity, but may be used to ascertain degrees of functional disability and levels of surgical risk. A $\dot{V}_{O_2}$ at the anaerobic threshold of less than 11 mL/min/kg has been found to significantly increase mortality risk for major surgery in the elderly. Current NICE guidelines suggest that a $\dot{V}_{O_2\,\text{PEAK}}$ of less than 15 mL/min/kg indicates increased risk of mortality for lung cancer surgery.

Table 15.2 Characteristic patterns of change during CPET in the major categories of exercise limiting disease

	Airway disease	Restrictive disease	Ischemic heart disease	Cardiomyopathy	Pulmonary vascular disease
Peak heart rate	↓	→	↔	↔	↔
Breathing reserve	↓	↓ (with ↑ RR)	↔ or ↑	↔ or ↑	↔ or ↑
$\Delta \dot{V}_{O_2}/\Delta WR$ slope	↔/↓	↔/↓	↔ then ↓	→	→
ECG changes	No	No	S–T ↓	No	No
$HR/\dot{V}_{O_2}$ slope	↔	↔	↔ then ↑	↑	↔
O_2 pulse	Rises but ↓peak	Rises but ↓peak	early and ↓ peak, then may decline ±↑Post ex	May be flat ↓peak ↑post Ex	Flat ↓peak
$\dot{V}_E/\dot{V}_{CO_2}$ @ AT	↑	↑	↔	↑	↑
S_pO_2	↓	↓	↔	↔	↓

SPECIFIC CONSIDERATIONS

CPET is demanding of resources, so careful consideration should be given to appropriate referral. Contraindications should be carefully evaluated due to the risks involved, and the mode of exercise available should be appropriate and achievable for the patient concerned.

KEY POINTS/SUMMARY

- CPET is useful to help identify the system responsible for exercise intolerance and/or dyspnoea in cases where resting assessments of cardiovascular and pulmonary function are unhelpful or equivocal. CPET can also quantify physiological functional status for disability or pre-surgical assessment, and evaluate the efficacy of medical interventions.
- A reduced breathing reserve at peak exercise is a cardinal feature of those whose respiratory function limits exercise tolerance. This may often be accompanied by arterial oxygen desaturation, particularly in interstitial lung disease or pulmonary vasculopathy, due to ventilation–perfusion mismatch.
- A disproportionately high HR response during all or part of an incremental exercise test is a distinguishing feature of most myocardial causes of exercise intolerance. This is usually not accompanied by arterial oxygen desaturation, except in advanced severe disease, which would usually preclude such a test.
- Pulmonary vascular disorders are characterised by a disproportionately high ventilatory response to exercise, flat oxygen pulse, and profound arterial oxygen desaturation.

PART ④

INTERPRETATION

16

A strategy for interpretation of pulmonary function tests

INTRODUCTION

The following strategy offers an approach to medical interpretation of a set of lung function data. In practical terms, interpretation of the data is guided heavily by the clinician's first impression of the patient, and the suspected diagnosis. In producing this scheme, it is not possible to recapitulate all of the nuances of data interpretation discussed in the preceding text. Therefore, it should be read in conjunction with the relevant chapters. Figure 16.1 presents this algorithm as a flowchart.

STEP 1 – IS THERE EVIDENCE OF OBSTRUCTION?

Is the shape of the flow–volume loop normal? Look for:

- Scalloping of the descending arm of the expiratory curve, indicative of obstruction.
- Loss of the peaks of expiration or inspiration ('decapitation'), indicative of large airway obstruction.
- Reduction of the ratio of FEV_1/FVC or FEV_1/VC. (Use whichever of FVC or VC is greater in value for this calculation.) Ideally compare these ratios to standard residuals, or the lower limit of normality, otherwise take 0.7 as the cut-off (see 'Normal values' in Chapter 3).

No

There is no evidence of obstruction on present evidence. Go to Step 2.

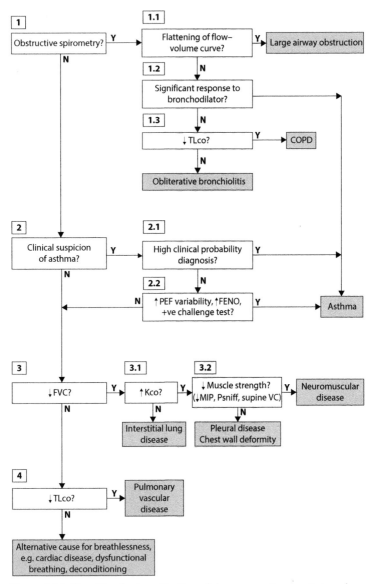

Figure 16.1 Algorithm for investigation of dyspnoea using respiratory function tests including useful clinical considerations.

Yes

An obstructive defect is present, suggestive of airway disease, possibly caused by chronic obstructive pulmonary disease (COPD), asthma, bronchiectasis or rarely, large airway obstruction or obliterative bronchiolitis. Go to Step 1.1 to differentiate, if the answer is not already clear from the clinical findings.

STEP 1.1 – IS THERE ANY FLATTENING/DECAPITATION OF THE FLOW–VOLUME CURVE?
Are there any findings to suggest large airway obstruction?

No

The flow–volume loop appears obstructed, but without any suggestion of large airway obstruction. Go to Step 1.2.

Yes

Suspect large airway obstruction. Is there any sign of stridor on examination? Is a mediastinal mass visible on the chest x-ray? Consider computed tomography (CT) followed by bronchoscopy. Patients with large airway obstruction are prone to sudden deterioration, so some urgency may be required, depending upon the time course of events and severity of obstruction. Stridor is an ominous sign.

STEP 1.2 – ADMINISTRATION OF BRONCHODILATOR
Is there a significant response to administration of a bronchodilator?

Yes

If the FEV_1 ratio is normalised following administration of bronchodilator, COPD is excluded and the findings are consistent with a diagnosis of asthma. Asthma is also likely if bronchodilator causes significant improvement in FEV_1 (>400 mL), even though the value may remain below the normal range (see 'Reversibility' in Chapter 4).

No

If an obstructive defect persists without significant response to bronchodilator, then a cause of fixed airway obstruction should be sought, e.g. COPD, bronchiectasis or obliterative bronchiolitis. A significant smoking history e.g. >40 pack-years and age >50 suggests a diagnosis of COPD, under which circumstances it may be that no further tests are necessary to make a diagnosis.

High-volume chronic sputum production and susceptibility to chest infections are suggestive of bronchiectasis. Obliterative bronchiolitis is uncommon, but may be associated with connective-tissue disease, e.g. rheumatoid and occurs following organ transplant.

If further clarification is needed, go to Step 1.3.

STEP 1.3 – MEASURE TL_{CO}

Is TL_{CO} reduced?

No

TL_{CO} is preserved in cases of obliterative bronchiolitis. TL_{CO} is also preserved in patients with asthma, even though airway obstruction may become fixed in chronic asthmatics. Go to Step 2, if needed, to distinguish.

Yes

The combination of an obstructive defect and reduction of TLco is consistent with a diagnosis of COPD (or possibly bronchiectasis, if suggested by the history).

STEP 2 – IS THERE A CLINICAL SUSPICION OF ASTHMA?

Is asthma a possible diagnosis, from the history or examination findings? Normal spirometry does not exclude a diagnosis of asthma, if measured when a patient is asymptomatic, although normal spirometry when symptomatic would make asthma an unlikely cause of the symptoms.

No

If nothing supports a diagnosis of asthma go to Step 3. The possibility of asthma can be revisited if other investigations are unhelpful, or if new clinical information becomes available.

Yes

Go to Step 2.1

STEP 2.1 – CAN YOU MAKE A HIGH PROBABILITY CLINICAL DIAGNOSIS OF ASTHMA?

Most cases of asthma may be diagnosed from the history of wheeze, chest tightness, dyspnoea, or cough, any of which may be worse at night or in the early mornings, on exercise or after exposure to allergens.

On the basis of the above, can you make a high probability clinical diagnosis?

No

There is an intermediate probability diagnosis of asthma. Go to Step 2.2.

Yes

Diagnose asthma. Make a trial of treatment.

STEP 2.2 – DO AIRWAY INVESTIGATIONS SUPPORT A DIAGNOSIS OF ASTHMA?

An uncertain diagnosis of asthma may be supported by a variety of tests:

- Consider a period of peak flow monitoring, to detect variability. The sensitivity of this test is quite low, but it may be a reasonable measure in primary care or in the absence of more sophisticated investigations. Is there significant diurnal variability (10%) on twice daily monitoring? (see 'Peak flow variability in the diagnosis of asthma' in Chapter 2).
- Measurement of fractional concentration of expired nitric oxide (Fe_{NO}) may be helpful if positive at a level of >50 ppb. Some individuals without asthma may register positive results, but the higher the reading the more specific the result becomes. Note that Fe_{NO} may not be elevated in patients with non-eosinophilic asthma phenotypes nor smokers (see Chapter 5).
- Administration of bronchodilator would probably not evoke a positive response in those with normal baseline spirometry, so this test would add little at this point.
- Finally, a negative bronchial challenge test virtually excludes a diagnosis of asthma (see 'Challenge testing' in Chapter 4).
- A trial of treatment with inhaled corticosteroid which brings an improvement in FEV_1 >400 mL would confirm a diagnosis of asthma.

No

Asthma is unlikely, proceed to Step 3.

Yes

Diagnose asthma and implement a trial of treatment.

STEP 3 – IS THE FVC REDUCED?

Are either of the FVC or VC abnormal? (Use whichever is greater in value.)

No

A restrictive defect is unlikely (though occasionally total lung capacity (TLC) may be reduced, despite preservation of VC – see 'Patterns of abnormality' in Chapter 7). Proceed to Step 4.

Yes

There may be a restrictive defect. It may be helpful to measure static lung volumes, as confirmation of a restrictive defect hinges upon demonstration of a low TLC. However, gas transfer data are often more discriminative. Go to Step 3.1.

STEP 3.1 – MEASURE GAS TRANSFER

Is the K_{CO} raised?

No

There is a reduction of FVC, with a K_{CO} which is normal or impaired. Suspect interstitial lung disease (ILD). TL_{CO} should also be examined, as reduction of TL_{CO} is more sensitive in detection of abnormality than reduction in K_{CO}. Fine inspiratory crepitations are usually present on auscultation, though they may be absent in patients with sarcoidosis. Are there any risk factors for ILD e.g. connective-tissue disease, antigen or occupational exposure, treatment with drugs known to cause pulmonary toxicity? Consider a high-resolution CT scan of the thorax.

Yes

A raised K_{CO} may be seen in cases of extra-pulmonary restriction, possibly due to chest wall, pleural, or neuromuscular disease (see 'Patterns of abnormality' in Chapter 6).

Note that K_{CO} may occasionally be greater than predicted early in the course of ILD, if it causes a discrete loss of units (see 'Discrete loss of lung units' in Chapter 6). However, any elevation of K_{CO} is modest under such circumstances and K_{CO} would fall within the normal range, even if somewhat greater than predicted (see Chapter 1). Consider ILD, but if it seems unlikely then go to Step 3.2.

Elevation of TL$_{CO}$ and K$_{CO}$ also occurs in alveolar haemorrhage, although these patients are often too unwell to complete pulmonary function testing, and the window of opportunity to identify acute pulmonary haemorrhage by measurement of TL$_{CO}$ is often short. In cases of alveolar haemorrhage, the chest x-ray is always dramatically abnormal. Note that performing the forced inspiratory and expiratory manoeuvres which are necessary for measurement of spirometry may be unwise in patients with haemoptysis.

STEP 3.2 – EVALUATE RESPIRATORY MUSCLE STRENGTH

A normal supine VC effectively excludes clinically significant muscle weakness. A significant drop in the VC from upright to supine is highly suspicious for muscle weakness, in which case no further pulmonary function tests may be needed. However, if there is an indeterminate drop in supine VC, further investigation is required, with maximum inspiratory and expiratory pressures (MIP and MEP) and/or nasal sniff pressure.

Is there significant abnormality of supine VC, MIP, MEP, or nasal sniff pressure?

Yes

Respiratory muscle weakness is confirmed. Measure creatine kinase (CK) and arterial blood gases, consider electromyogram (EMG) and sleep study. Seek neurological advice.

No

The findings suggest extra-pulmonary restriction, but without evidence of muscle weakness. Consider other causes of extra-pulmonary restriction such as pleural disease or chest wall abnormality such as scoliosis or ankylosing spondylitis. Measure TLC to confirm a restrictive state if none of the above appear to be present. Consider a CT scan of the thorax.

STEP 4 – IS TL$_{CO}$ REDUCED?

Yes

If spirometry and the chest x-ray are normal, despite reduced TL$_{CO}$, suspect pulmonary vascular disease. Consider performing a CT pulmonary angiogram or perfusion scan to exclude pulmonary embolism.

Marked reduction of TL$_{CO}$ may also occur despite preservation of spirometry in cases where emphysema and pulmonary fibrosis coexist. The chest x-ray would be abnormal in such cases.

No

No abnormality has been detected.

The combination of normal spirometry and gas transfer practically excludes respiratory disease as a cause of dyspnoea, and an alternative aetiology should be sought. Dysfunctional breathing and deconditioning are both common causes of perceived dyspnoea. Consider cardiologic investigations if appropriate. If doubt remains, consider cardiopulmonary exercise testing (CPET).

17

Characteristic pulmonary function abnormalities

This chapter highlights the patterns of change in the major lung function indices for the most commonly encountered respiratory diseases. For simplicity, only the indices which would be expected to fall outside of the normal range are included.

AIRWAY DISEASES

ASTHMA

PEF and FEV_1 ratio	Reduced, if symptomatic when measured
FEV_1	Often reduced
Flow–volume loop	Concavity of expiratory curve
Reversibility	Present
sR_{aw}	Increased
RV and RV/TLC	Increased if gas trapping occurs
FE_{NO}	Increased in the eosinophilic phenotype
Challenge test	Invariably positive

CHRONIC OBSTRUCTIVE PULMONARY DISEASE

PEF and FEV_1 ratio	Reduced
FEV_1	Reduced in comparison to FVC
Flow–volume loop	Concavity of expiratory curve. 'Church steeple' appearance seen in advanced emphysema
Reversibility	Absent or incomplete; normalisation of spirometry not attainable
sR_{aw}	Increased
RV and RV/TLC	Increased if gas trapping occurs

TL_{CO} and K_{CO}	Reduced
ABG	Type 1 or 2 respiratory failure in those with advanced disease

BRONCHIOLITIS

PEF and FEV_1 ratio	Reduced
FEV_1	Reduced
Flow–volume loop	Concavity of expiratory curve or 'church steeple' appearance seen in advanced disease
RV and RV/TLC	Increased if gas trapping occurs
TL_{CO}	Preserved, until advanced disease, e.g. FEV_1 <1L

BRONCHIECTASIS

PEF and FEV_1 ratio	Reduced
FEV_1	Usually reduced
Flow–volume loop	Concavity of expiratory loop
RV and RV/TLC	Maybe increased if gas trapping occurs
TL_{CO} and K_{CO}	Often reduced

LARGE AIRWAY OBSTRUCTION – VARIABLE EXTRATHORACIC

PIF	Reduced
Flow–volume loop	Flattened appearance of inspiratory curve

LARGE AIRWAY OBSTRUCTION – VARIABLE INTRATHORACIC

PEF and FEV_1	Reduced (PEF reduced more than FEV_1)
Flow–volume loop	Square/rectangular flattened appearance of expiratory curve

FIXED UPPER AIRWAY OBSTRUCTION

FEV_1	Reduced
FEV_1 ratio	Reduced
PEF and PIF	Reduced
Flow–volume loop	Rectangular/flattened appearance of inspiratory and expiratory curve

RESTRICTIVE DISEASES

INTERSTITIAL LUNG DISEASE

FEV_1	Reduced
FEV_1 ratio	Normal and often increased
FVC	Reduced
TLC	Reduced
Flow–volume loop	Normal shape but reduced in magnitude or 'wizard's hat' appearance
RV	Normal or slightly reduced, so that RV/TLC usually increased
TL_{CO}, K_{CO}, and V_A	Reduced. TL_{CO} usually more reduced than K_{CO}
ABG	Arterial P_aO_2 may be normal initially. Alveolar–arterial P_aO_2 difference gradient increased
S_pO_2	Desaturation on exercise common

PLEURAL DISEASE (WITH NO ACCOMPANYING INTERSTITIAL INVOLVEMENT)

FEV_1	Reduced
FVC	Reduced
Flow–volume loop	Normal shape but reduced in magnitude
TLC	Reduced
TL_{CO} and V_A	Reduced
K_{CO}	Increased

CHEST WALL DEFORMITY

FEV_1	Reduced
FVC	Reduced
Flow–volume loop	Normal shape but reduced in magnitude
TLC	Reduced
RV	May be increased
TL_{CO} and V_A	Reduced
K_{CO}	Increased

MUSCLE WEAKNESS

FEV_1 and PEF	Reduced
FVC	Reduced
Flow–volume loop	Reduced in magnitude, often with a poor expiratory peak and early end to expiration
TLC	Reduced
RV	Increased
RV/TLC	Increased
Postural change	Often >15% drop in vital capacity in supine position with diaphragmatic weakness or paralysis
TL_{CO} and V_A	Reduced
K_{CO}	Increased
ABG	Type 2 respiratory failure occurs late; CO_2 may be raised in the morning
A–a P_aO_2 gradient	Usually normal

POST-PULMONARY RESECTION SURGERY (E.G. LOBECTOMY, PNEUMONECTOMY)

FEV_1, PEF, and FVC	Reduced, but by less than the percentage of lung resection
RV	Reduced
TL_{CO} and V_A	Reduced
K_{CO}	Increased

PULMONARY VASCULAR DISEASE

PULMONARY ARTERIAL HYPERTENSION

TL_{CO} and K_{CO}	Reduced equally
S_pO_2	Reduced at rest in advanced disease. Profound desaturation on exercise

RECURRENT PULMONARY EMBOLI

TL_{CO}	Low or normal
K_{CO}	Low or normal
ABG	P_aO_2 reduced, with increased A–a P_{O_2} gradient
S_pO_2	Reduced at rest in advanced disease. Desaturation on exercise

CHRONIC PULMONARY VENOUS CONGESTION

TLC	Reduced
RV	Increased
TL_{CO} and K_{CO}	Reduced

CARBON MONOXIDE POISONING

S_pO_2	Spuriously normal
Directly measured S_aO_2	Reduced
P_aO_2	Normal
Carboxyhaemoglobin	Raised

Table 17.1 provides a summary of the characteristic abnormalities seen in the most commonly pulmonary disorders.

Table 17.1 Changes to major lung function indices with disease

Index	Asthma	COPD	ILD	Muscle weakness	PAH
FEV_1	↓ or ↔	↓	↓	↓	↔
FVC	↔ or ↓	↔ or ↓	↓	↓	↔
FEV_1 ratio	↓	↓	**↑ or ↔**	↔	↔
TLC	↑	↑	↓	↓	↔
RV	↑	↑	↔ or ↓	↑	↔
RV/TLC	↑	↑	↔ or ↑	↑	
TL_{CO}	↔	↓	↓	↓	↓
V_A	↔	↔	↓	↓	↔
K_{CO}	↔	↓	↓	↑	↓

Note: The patterns of abnormality are unique. Discriminative indices are indicted in bold. Although not every case exhibits the typical abnormality, the pattern of change may point to the aetiology.

References

1. Pellegrino R, Viegi G, Brusasco V, et al. Interpretative strategies for lung function tests. *Eur Respir J* 2005;**26**(5):948–68.
2. Gregg I, Nunn AJ. Peak expiratory flow in normal subjects. *Br Med J* 1973;**3**(5874):282–4.
3. Quanjer PH, Tammeling GJ, Cotes JE, et al. Lung volumes and forced ventilatory flows. Report Working Party Standardization of Lung Function Tests, European Community for Steel and Coal. Official Statement of the European Respiratory Society. *Eur Respir J Suppl* 1993;**16**:5–40.
4. British Thoracic Society, Scottish Intercollegiate Guidelines Network. British guideline on the management of asthma. A national clinical guideline. 2016. ISBN 978 1 909103 47 4. Scottish Intercollegiate Guidelines Network, Edinburgh.
5. Cooper BG. An update on contraindications for lung function testing. *Thorax* 2011;**66**(8):714–23.
6. American Association for Respiratory Care. AARC Clinical Practice Guideline. Spirometry, 1996 update. *Respir Care* 1996;**41**(7):629–36.
7. Morris DG, Sheppard D. Pulmonary emphysema: When more is less. *Physiology (Bethesda)* 2006;**21**:396–403.
8. Global Initiative for Chronic Obstructive Lung Disease. Global Strategy for the Diagnosis, Management, and Prevention of COPD, 2016. Available from http://goldcopd.org/global-strategy-diagnosis-management-prevention-copd-2016/. Accessed 2016.
9. National Institute for Health and Care Excellence. Chronic obstructive pulmonary disease in over 16's: diagnosis and management. Available from http://nice.org.uk/guidance/cg101
10. Pulmonaria Group. SpirXpert (cited 2016). Available from: http://www.spirxpert.com/index.html.
11. Global Initiative for Asthma. Global Strategy for Asthma Management and Prevention. 2015.

12. Dykstra BJ, Scanlon PD, Kester MM, et al. Lung volumes in 4,774 patients with obstructive lung disease. *Chest* 1999;**115**(1):68–74.

13. Hyatt RE, Scanlon PD, Nakamura M. *Interpretation of Pulmonary Function Tests*, 4th edition. Philadelphia, PA: Lippincott Williams and Wilkins, 2014.

14. Kannel WB, Hubert H, Lew EA. Vital capacity as a predictor of cardiovascular disease: The Framingham study. *Am Heart J* 1983;**105**(2):311–5.

15. Holleman DR, Jr., Simel DL. Does the clinical examination predict airflow limitation? *JAMA* 1995;**273**(4):313–9.

16. Crapo RO, Casaburi R, Coates AL, et al. Guidelines for methacholine and exercise challenge testing-1999. This official statement of the American Thoracic Society was adopted by the ATS Board of Directors, July 1999. *Am J Respir Crit Care Med* 2000;**161**(1):309–29.

17. Sterk PJ, Fabbri LM, Quanjer PH, et al. Airway responsiveness. Standardized challenge testing with pharmacological, physical and sensitizing stimuli in adults. Report working party standardization of lung function tests, European community for steel and coal. Official statement of the European respiratory society. *Eur Respir J Suppl* 1993;**16**:53–83.

18. Newton MF, O'Donnell DE, Forkert L. Response of lung volumes to inhaled salbutamol in a large population of patients with severe hyperinflation. *Chest* 2002;**121**(4):1042–50.

19. American Thoracic Society, European Respiratory Society. ATS/ERS recommendations for standardized procedures for the online and offline measurement of exhaled lower respiratory nitric oxide and nasal nitric oxide, 2005. *Am J Respir Crit Care Med* 2005;**171**(8):912–30.

20. Dweik RA, Boggs PB, Erzurum SC, et al. An official ATS clinical practice guideline: Interpretation of exhaled nitric oxide levels ($F_{E_{NO}}$) for clinical applications. *Am J Respir Crit Care Med* 2011;**184**(5):602–15.

21. Hughes JM, Pride NB. Examination of the carbon monoxide diffusing capacity (DLCO) in relation to its KCO and VA components. *Am J Respir Crit Care Med* 2012;**186**(2):132–9.

22. Gibson G. Lung volumes and elasticity. In: Hughes J, Pride N, eds. *Lung Function Tests Physiological Principles and Clinical Applications*, 1st edition. London: WB Saunders, 1999, pp. 45–57.

23. Aaron SD, Dales RE, Cardinal P. How accurate is spirometry at predicting restrictive pulmonary impairment? *Chest* 1999;**115**(3):869–73.

24. Casanova C, Cote C, de Torres JP, et al. Inspiratory-to-total lung capacity ratio predicts mortality in patients with chronic obstructive pulmonary disease. *Am J Respir Crit Care Med* 2005;**171**(6):591–7.

25. Mottram CD. *Ruppel's Manual of Pulmonary Function Testing*, 11th edition. St Louis, MO: Elsevier, 2017.

26. Oostveen E, MacLeod D, Lorino H, et al. ERS Task Force on Respiratory Impedance Measurements. The forced oscillation technique in clinical practice: Methodology, recommendations and future developments. *Eur Respir J* 2003;**22**:1026–41.

27. Allen SM, Hunt B, Green M. Fall in vital capacity with posture. *Br J Dis Chest* 1985;**79**(3):267–71.

28. Steier J, Kaul S, Seymour J, et al. The value of multiple tests of respiratory muscle strength. *Thorax* 2007;**62**(11):975–80.

29. Ragette R, Mellies U, Schwake C, et al. Patterns and predictors of sleep disordered breathing in primary myopathies. *Thorax* 2002;**57**(8):724–8.

30. Berry R, Brooks R, Gamaldo CE et al. for the American Academy of Sleep Medicine *The AASM Manual for the Scoring of Sleep and Associated Events: Rules, Terminology and Technical Specifications*, Version 2. 3. Darien, IL: American Academy of Sleep Medicine 2015.

31. Dohna-Schwake C, Ragette R, Teschler H, et al. Predictors of severe chest infections in pediatric neuromuscular disorders. *Neuromuscul Disord* 2006;**16**(5):325–8.

32. Lyall RA, Donaldson N, Polkey MI, et al. Respiratory muscle strength and ventilatory failure in amyotrophic lateral sclerosis. *Brain* 2001;**124**(Pt 10):2000–13.

33. Morgan RK, McNally S, Alexander M, et al. Use of Sniff nasal-inspiratory force to predict survival in amyotrophic lateral sclerosis. *Am J Respir Crit Care Med* 2005;**171**(3):269–74.

34. Hull J, Aniapravan R, Chan E, et al. British Thoracic Society guideline for respiratory management of children with neuromuscular weakness. *Thorax* 2012;**67**(Suppl. 1):i1–i40.

35. Szeinberg A, Tabachnik E, Rashed N, et al. Cough capacity in patients with muscular dystrophy. *Chest* 1988;**94**(6):1232–5.

36. Estenne M, De Troyer A. Mechanism of the postural dependence of vital capacity in tetraplegic subjects. *Am Rev Respir Dis* 1987;**135**(2):367–71.

37. Lim BL, Kelly AM. A meta-analysis on the utility of peripheral venous blood gas analyses in exacerbations of chronic obstructive pulmonary disease in the emergency department. *Eur J Emerg Med* 2010;**17**(5):246–8.

38. Crossley DJ, McGuire GP, Barrow PM, et al. Influence of inspired oxygen concentration on deadspace, respiratory drive, and $PaCO_2$ in intubated patients with chronic obstructive pulmonary disease. *Crit Care Med* 1997;**25**(9):1522–6.

39. Davidson AC, Banham S, Elliott M, et al. BTS/ICS guideline for the ventilatory management of acute hypercapnic respiratory failure in adults. *Thorax* 2016;**71**(Suppl. 2):ii1–ii35.

40. Van de Louw A, Cracco C, Cerf C, et al. Accuracy of pulse oximetry in the intensive care unit. *Intensive Care Med* 2001;**27**(10):1606–13.

41. McKeever TM, Hearson G, Housley G, et al. Using venous blood gas analysis in the assessment of COPD exacerbations: A prospective cohort study. *Thorax* 2016;**71**(3):210–5.

42. Hardinge M, Annandale J, Bourne S, et al. British Thoracic Society guidelines for home oxygen use in adults. *Thorax* 2015;**70**(Suppl. 1):i1–i43.

43. Zavorsky GS, Cao J, Mayo NE, et al. Arterial versus capillary blood gases: A meta-analysis. *Respir Physiol Neurobiol* 2007;**155**(3):268–79.

44. Eaton T, Rudkin S, Garrett JE. The clinical utility of arterialized ear-lobe capillary blood in the assessment of patients for long-term oxygen therapy. *Respir Med* 2001;**95**(8):655–60.

45. Lumb *AB. Nunn's Applied Respiratory Physiology*, 8th edition. London: Elsevier, 2016.

46. Brandis K. Acid-base physiology (updated 30 August 2015). Available from: http://www.anaesthesiaMCQ.com.

47. Graham T. Acid base online tutorial 2006 (cited 2016). Available from: http://fitsweb.uchc.edu/student/selectives/TimurGraham/Welcome.html.

48. Holland AE, Spruit MA, Troosters T, et al. An official European Respiratory Society/American Thoracic Society technical standard: Field walking tests in chronic respiratory disease. *Eur Respir J* 2014;**44**(6):1428–46.

49. ATS Committee on Proficiency Standards for Clinical Pulmonary Function Laboratories. ATS statement: Guidelines for the six-minute walk test. *Am J Respir Crit Care Med* 2002;**166**(1):111–7.

50. Casanova C, Celli BR, Barria P, et al. The 6-min walk distance in healthy subjects: Reference standards from seven countries. *Eur Respir J* 2011;**37**(1):150–6.

51. Probst VS, Hernandes NA, Teixeira DC, et al. Reference values for the incremental shuttle walking test. *Respir Med* 2012;**106**(2):243–8.

52. Celli BR, Cote CG, Marin JM, et al. The body-mass index, airflow obstruction, dyspnea, and exercise capacity index in chronic obstructive pulmonary disease. *N Engl J Med* 2004;**350**(10):1005–12.

53. Wasserman K. Diagnosing cardiovascular and lung pathophysiology from exercise gas exchange. *Chest* 1997;**112**(4):1091–101.

54. Older P, Hall A, Hader R. Cardiopulmonary exercise testing as a screening test for perioperative management of major surgery in the elderly. *Chest* 1999;**116**(2):355–62.

55. Tanaka H, Monahan KD, Seals DR. Age-predicted maximal heart rate revisited. *J Am Coll Cardiol* 2001;**37**(1):153–6.

FURTHER READING

GENERAL RESPIRATORY PHYSIOLOGY

Lumb A. *Nunn's Applied Respiratory Physiology*, 8th edition. London: Elsevier, 2017.

West JB. *West's Respiratory Physiology: The Essentials*, 10th edition. Baltimore, MD: Lippincott Williams and Wilkins, 2015.

RESPIRATORY MEDICINE/PATHOPHYSIOLOGY

Chapman S, Robinson G, Stradling J, West S, Wrightson J. *Oxford Handbook of Respiratory Medicine (Oxford Medical Handbooks)*, 3rd edition. London: Oxford University Press, 2014.

West JB. *Pulmonary Pathophysiology: The Essentials*, 10th edition. Baltimore, MD: Lippincott Williams and Wilkins, 2015.

REFERENCE VALUES

Quanjer PH, Stanojevic S, Cole TJ, et al. Multi-ethnic reference values for spirometry for the 3–95-yr age range: The global lung function 2012 equations. *Eur Respir J* 2012;**40**:1324–43.

GENERAL LUNG FUNCTION

British Thoracic Society. Guidelines for the measurement of respiratory function. *Respir Med* 1994;**88**:165–94.

Brusasco V, Crapo R, Viegi G, eds. ATS/ERS task force: Standardisation of lung function testing. General considerations for lung function testing. *Eur Respir J* 2005;**26**:153–61.

Cooper B, Evans A, Kendrick A, Newall C, (eds). *The ARTP Practical Handbook of Respiratory Function Testing – Parts 1 and 2*. Boldmere: Association for Respiratory Technology and Physiology, 2003.

Cotes JE, Chinn DJ, Miller MR. *Lung Function: Physiology, Measurement and Application in Medicine*, 6th edition. Oxford: Wiley-Blackwell, 2006.

Gibson GJ. *Clinical Tests of Respiratory Function*, 3rd edition. London: Hodder Arnold, 2008.

Hughes JMB. *Physiology and Practice of Pulmonary Function*. Boldmere: Association for Respiratory Technology and Physiology, 2009.

Hyatt RE, Scanlon PD. *Interpretation of Pulmonary Function Tests: A Practical Guide*, 3rd edition. Baltimore, MD: Lippincott Williams and Wilkins, 2008.

Mottram C. *Ruppel's Manual of Pulmonary Function Testing*, 10th edition. St. Louis, MO: Mosby Elsevier, 2012.

SPIROMETRY

Brusasco V, Crapo R, Viegi G, eds. ATS/ERS task force: Standardisation of lung function testing—Standardisation of spirometry. *Eur Respir J* 2005;**26**:319–38.

GAS TRANSFER

Brusasco V, Crapo R, Viegi G, eds. ATS/ERS task force: Standardisation of lung function testing. Standardisation of the single-breath determination of carbon monoxide uptake in the lung. *Eur Respir J* 2005;**26**:720–35.

Fitting JW. Transfer factor for carbon monoxide: A glance behind the scene. *Swiss Med Wkly* 2004;**134**:413–8.

LUNG VOLUMES

Brusasco V, Crapo R, Viegi G, eds. ATS/ERS task force: Standardisation of lung function testing. Standardisation of the measurement of lung volumes. *Eur Respir J* 2005;**26**:511–22.

CHALLENGE TESTING

ERS Task Force. Indirect airway challenges. *Eur Respir J* 2003;**21**:1050–68.

RESPIRATORY MUSCLE FUNCTION

American Thoracic Society/European Respiratory Society. ATS/ERS statement on respiratory muscle testing. *Am J Respir Crit Care Med* *2002*;166:518–624.

FIELD EXERCISE TESTS

Singh SJ, Puhan MA, Andrianopoulos V, et al. An official systematic review of the European Respiratory Society/American Thoracic Society: Measurement properties of field walking tests in chronic respiratory disease. *Eur Respir J* 2014;**44**:1447–78.

CARDIOPULMONARY EXERCISE TESTS

American College of Sports Medicine. *ACSM's Guidelines for Exercise Testing and Prescription*, 9th edition. Baltimore, MD: Lippincott Williams and Wilkins, 2013.

American Thoracic Society, American College of Chest Physicians. ATS/ACCP Statement on cardiopulmonary exercise testing. *Am J Respir Crit Care Med* 2003;**167**:211–77.

Astrand P-O, Rodahl K, Dahl HA, Stromme SB. *Textbook of Work Physiology*, 4th edition. Champaign, IL: Human Kinetics, 2003.

Balady GJ, Arena R, Sietsema K, et al. Clinician's guide to cardiopulmonary exercise testing in adults: A scientific statement from the American Heart Association. *Circulation* 2010;**122**:191–225.

Roca J, Whipp BJ, Agustí AGN, et al. Clinical exercise testing with reference to lung diseases: indications, standardization and interpretation strategies. ERS Task Force on Standardization of Clinical Exercise Testing. *Eur Respir J* 1997;**10**:2662–89.

Cooper CB, Storer TW. *Exercise Testing and Interpretation: A Practical Approach*. Cambridge: Cambridge University Press, 2004.

ERS Task Force. Recommendations on the use of exercise testing in clinical practice. *Eur Respir J* 2007;**29**:185–209.

Wasserman K, Hansen J, Sietsema K, et al. *Principles of Exercise Testing and Interpretation: Including Pathophysiology and Clinical Applications*, 5th edition. Baltimore, MD: Lippincott Williams and Wilkins, 2011.

Index